LARGE PRINT EDITION

LOW VISION MATTERS

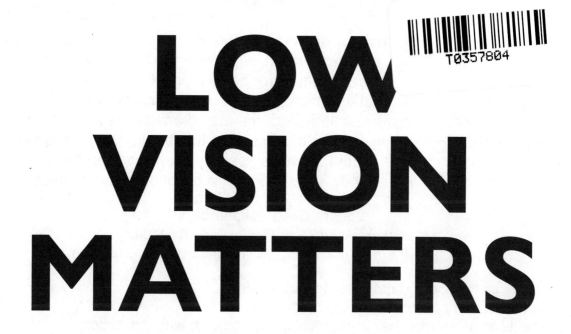

A PRACTICAL GUIDE TO LIVING WITH LOW VISION & BLINDNESS

LAURA J. STEVENS, MSci
THOMAS BLACKMAN, MHA

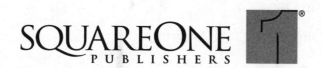

SQUAREONE
PUBLISHERS

EDITOR: Anthony Pomes
COVER DESIGN/TYPESETTING: Gary A. Rosenberg

The information and advice contained in this book are based upon the research and the personal and professional experiences of the authors. They are not intended as a substitute for consulting with an eye care professional. The publisher and authors are not responsible for any adverse effects or consequences resulting from the use of any of the suggestions, procedures, or use of equipment discussed in this book. All matters pertaining to your eyecare should be supervised by a eye care professional. It is a sign of wisdom, not cowardice, to seek a second or third opinion.

Square One Publishers

115 Herricks Road • Garden City Park, NY 11040
(516) 535-2010 • (877) 900-BOOK • www.squareonepublishers.com

Library of Congress Cataloging-in-Publication
Names: Stevens, Laura J., 1945– author.
Title: Low vision matters : a practical guide to living with low vision
   & blindness / Laura Stevens, MSci, Thomas Blackman, MHA.
Description: Garden City Park, NY : Square One Publishers, 2025. |
   Includes index.
Identifiers: LCCN 2024025627 | ISBN 9780757005343 (paperback) |
   ISBN 9780757055348 (ebook)
Subjects: LCSH: Self-help techniques. | Low vision. | Blindness.
Classification: LCC BF632 .S742 2024 | DDC 646.70087/1—dc23/
eng/20240703
LC record available at https://lccn.loc.gov/2024025627

ISBN 978-0-7570-0534-3 (pb) ISBN 978-0-7570-5534-8 (eb)

Copyright © 2025 by Laura Stevens and Thomas Blackman

All rights reserved. No part of this publication may be reproduced, stored in a retrieval system, or transmitted, in any form or by any means, electronic, mechanical, photocopying, recording, or otherwise, without the prior written permission of the publisher. Furthermore, no existing portions of the copyrighted material contained herein shall be repurposed or drawn upon by any/all present or future forms of AI (artificial intelligence) systems/applications worldwide.

Printed in the United States of America

10 9 8 7 6 5 4 3 2 1

Contents

PART 2 PRODUCTS AND THEIR FEATURES

To my beloved mother,
Flora E. Stoner
—LS

To my wife, Jenny,
for her support and contributions
—TB

Credits

Photographs on pages 121, 122, 204, 208, 210, 212, 220, 238, 241, 243, 244, 247, and 252 reprinted by permission of Vispero.

Photographs on pages 66, 69, 79, 97, 123, 125, 142, 199, 206, 235, 289, and 291 reprinted by permission of LS&S, LLC.

Image on page 144 courtesy of Mastercard International Incorporated.

Illustration on page 171 reprinted courtesy of the U.S. Department of Agriculture.

Photographs on page 201 reprinted by permission of WeWALK Limited.

Acknowledgments

I want to thank many important people who helped make this book possible. First, my family members—my parents who always encouraged me to undertake new projects, and especially my mother, whose own severe vision loss occurred many years ago—for inspiring me to write this book. Also, my beloved husband, George E. Stevens, a professor of journalism, who greatly improved anything I wrote and encouraged me to write my first books in the 1970s; and my dear sons, Jack and Jeff, who support and encourage me each day in every way.

I'd also like to thank all my friends—especially Dorothy Boyce, Rosann Spitzer, Mary Campbell, Linda Pierret, and Judy Wright—who have always supported and encouraged me over the years. Also, my pastors, Tracey Leslie and Suzanne Clementz, who have helped me deal with my loss of vision and so much more. I'd also like to thank my dear friend Cathy Misner, who helps me deal with my vision loss in many practical ways. I am forever grateful to all of these wonderful friends.

I am also grateful to those who have encouraged my writing career, including Wiliam G. Crook and all the editors at Doubleday, Macmillan, and Random House and, in later years, Square One Publishers' Rudy Shur, who has helped and guided Tom Blackman and me every step of the way on this book. Many thanks also to those Square One editors who have made my writing sound coherent and professional, especially Michael Weatherhead and Anthony Pomes.

And finally, I want to thank my co-author, Tom Blackman, who has personally helped me with my vision challenges and has contributed greatly to all the technology information that has made this book possible.

—LS

I would like to take this opportunity to acknowledge and thank those who have helped me in my career, which then led to an opportunity to contribute to this project. My first job in Elkhart, Indiana in 1973 provided an opportunity to meet Mary and Ron Workman. Ron was totally blind and owned a very successful insurance business. He demonstrated to me that with the right support at the right time, one can set goals and be successful. Mary and Ron encouraged me to attend graduate school to work in this field.

After obtaining a Master's degree in Blind Rehabilitation in 1975, I was very fortunate to work over the years with many blind co-workers in Indiana who all had high standards for the services we delivered. Gene Riech, Marvin Price, James Michaels, Bill Powell, Kurt Diechmann, and Elnora Dillon were fantastic professionals with high standards.

Finally, thanks to Ms. Laura Stevens for inviting me to be a part of this book. Thanks also to Mr. Rudy Shur for his professional assistance in editing my content.

—TB

Preface

I was diagnosed with age-related macular degeneration (AMD) in 2013. AMD severely affects the center of your vision so you struggle to see things up close and at a distance. Although very disturbing, my diagnosis was not a complete surprise because my mother had severe vision loss due to AMD, and I knew that genes play a major role.

My life is so much better than my mother's in several ways. In my mother's day, there was no way to learn about the disease. She depended upon her doctor for medical information. Contrast that with today where you can go online and find out all kinds of helpful information: the causes of the disease, risk factors, and new treatments. For example, today many eye doctors prescribe certain nutrients such as AREDS, a supplement sold over-the-counter at all pharmacies. The nutrients don't cure the disease but they can help slow the progress.

Also, doctors have new injectable drugs for both types of AMD, dry and wet. Again, these treatments do not cure the disease but can slow the progression. Because AMD is a disease of older persons and our population is aging, there is an amazing amount of ongoing research positioned to help us find better answers. My mother had none of those advantages.

In addition, my mother had no way to pursue her passions. She had always loved to read books and magazines. She had also studied music in her teens and loved all kinds of music. She enjoyed watching football, basketball, tennis, and golf, but she did not have a large TV. She lost her independence when she could no longer drive herself to the library, stores, or to have lunch with friends. She depended upon my father to take her wherever she needed to go.

With today's technology, I am able to listen to Alexa read any book or play any music I desire. I also have a very large TV so that I can follow sports. I even have a watch that tells me the time out loud. Using a car service to go to church, the store, or to visit friends helps me retain some sense of independence. These are just a few of the opportunities I have in today's world that my mother would have killed for.

In recent years, my vision declined, and I struggled to continue my profession of writing books about health issues. I met this book's co-author, Tom Blackman, a vision therapist who recommended a computer program to enlarge the print so I could continue to write. He also had many other tools to help me. So given that I was a writer and now had firsthand personal experience of vision loss, while Tom was a talented vision therapist, we teamed up to write this book.

—Laura Stevens

My goal in being a part of this book was to provide useful easy-to-understand information and current up-to-date resources in a single source provided in print, digital, or audio format. My hope is that this book will encourage those with low vision and blindness to remain independent, be encouraged, and be proactive. If each reader can find a resource and useful information, then I have accomplished my goal.

My interest in working in rehabilitation services for persons with vision loss began with my very first job upon graduating from college. That was back in 1973. The rehabilitation center where I worked had a small department dedicated to Orientation & Mobility, as well as Activities of Daily Living services. My interest led me to obtain a Master's degree in Blind Rehabilitation in 1975. This was the beginning of a career for me that has now spanned nearly fifty years.

During my career, the 1973 Rehabilitation Act and the 1990 Americans with Disabilities Act were milestones that helped lead to the development of the new field of Assistive Technology for persons with disabilities. Most of my work has been in this field. Much of our book is dedicated to assistive technology products, information, and services as well as many other topics. I hope you find this book helpful.

—Thomas Blackman

How to Read (or Listen) to This Book

We understand that reading this book—even though it is in large print—may be difficult for some of you. Because low vision ranges in severity—from mild to extreme—one reader may struggle while another has no problem. We understand that reading may take a lot of effort, sometimes leaving us frustrated and exhausted. If that is a problem for you, here are some suggestions as you start to read this book:

■ Pace yourself. You may be only able to read one chapter at one sitting, or even only a part of a chapter.

■ Review the "Table of Contents" to identify those chapters that look most helpful for your situation and start with them. You can always go back later to read the other chapters.

■ Within any given chapter, identify those sections that apply to you and skip the rest. We have tried to structure the book's chapters so that each section is independent of the others.

■ If the print of this book is not large enough for you, use a magnification device to enlarge the words, so you can see them better. There are handheld magnifiers, and magnifiers that can enlarge a whole page. You will learn more about your magnification options in some of the chapters.

■ Take the ebook edition of this book and store it on your computer or tablet. Then enlarge the size of the text (font) to a size that you can read.

■ If you still struggle, consider ways to have this book read aloud. Using the ebook edition, transfer the file to your smartphone, tablet, or computer. Once done, go into your device's settings to enable the device to read the copy on your screen aloud to you.

At this point, you may need to read Chapters 2 and 13 to learn more about magnification devices, enlarging print, or enabling a "read aloud" setting on your smartphone, tablet, or computer. If it is still an issue, you may want to ask someone who has some tech skills to help you—a relative, friend, or neighbor.

Finally, it's important that you find for yourself the *easiest* way to read this book. We think the information it contains will greatly improve the quality of your life. So be patient with yourself until you learn these new skills. You can do this!

Introduction

Low vision is defined as the inability to see things clearly, close up and at a distance, even with the aid of glasses or contacts. There are a number of reasons why this happens. For some, medical conditions, surgical procedures and/or medications can improve their vision. However, for others, their medical options are limited, and over time, their eyesight may worsen.

In the past, low vision truly limited an individual's ability to live a normal life. Everyday tasks were either difficult or impossible to do. For most, people with low vision found themselves dependent on others to get through each day. However, as you will read—or listen to—things have changed greatly.

In 1990, a major step was taken with the passage of the Americans with Disabilities Act. Initially, it prohibited discrimination against individuals with disabilities in all areas of public life, including jobs, schools, transportation, and all public and private places that are open to the general public, but it did more. It also set guidelines for companies to provide special services

1

to those with disabilities—such as poor or no vision—which you may not be aware of.

Perhaps even more important is the technological breakthroughs that have occurred over the last decade. Where once these high-tech services were found only in works of science fiction, today they are actually available for use in your home, outdoors, and at work.

If you are a person with low vision, or if you are reading this book on behalf of another person, it should come as no surprise to understand how challenging this condition can be. At the same time, it is the aim of this book to provide as complete an overview of what products and services are available to assist those people with poor vision, as well as blindness. As you will learn, there are many free services available to help. There are also a wide range of technological equipment and services that can be somewhat pricey. It is important to shop around to get the best dollar values or find a program that can help with the cost.

Two of the game changers for people with poor vision are smartphones and voice-activated devices (such as those using Alexa and Siri). It is natural that there is going to be a learning curve in their usage, but once a service has been installed and used several times, there will come a sense of newfound freedom.

This book is designed to cover all the essential parts of a person's life. It is divided into two parts. Part

1 focuses on the different aspects necessary to deal with low vision. It contains twelve chapters. Chapter 1 explains the importance of having the right support team in place. Chapter 2 discusses the various types of virtual assistance aids now available, covering both mobile and stationary devices. Chapter 3 offers information on making your home more secure. Chapter 4 details what can be done to prepare for possible emergency situations. Chapter 5 takes a look at what devices and software programs are available to improve the living condition within your home. Chapter 6 offers a number of suggestions to have fun in your home. Chapter 7 provides important advice when traveling outside of the home. Chapter 8 examines the various technologies to make writing and reading easier. Chapter 9 deals with finances, from paying bills to investing. Chapter 10 offers key information on maintaining your health and all that goes along with it. Chapter 11 presents information dealing with blindness. And the last chapter looks at today's many job opportunities

Part 2 contains five chapters; each focused on the types of products available for people with low vision and blindness. This includes magnification options, software reading programs, assistive home products, and medical devices. This is followed by an extensive *Resources* section, providing information on the organizations, services, manufacturers, and catalog companies that specialize in meeting the needs of those with low vision and blindness.

CONCLUSION

There is a great deal to learn as you go through this book. To some degree, it may seem overwhelming—whether it's having a network of friends and professionals to call on or it's making the house as safe to live in as possible. There is a lot to cover. And while each topic is important, we would suggest that you first focus on the areas that are most important to the person with low vision. It is only natural to want to remain as independent and secure as possible.

The world is truly different than it was just a decade ago. It is important to take advantage of the help that is out there. Be proactive and ask questions. Often, you will find there are different options to reach each goal. And yet, it is also important to understand that not everything works smoothly. There will likely be learning curves that will bring moments of frustration and anxiety. However, we sincerely hope the information in this book will help prepare you for what happens moving forward and that it opens the door to a better future.

PART 1

LIVING WITH LOW VISION

There is no question that low vision can greatly impact your daily life. The many things you took for granted, such as driving to visit a friend, working on your computer, reading a book, or going grocery shopping, become difficult tasks you must now learn to cope with. While you may have already developed many ways to deal with your low vision, today—given modern technology—there are a number of solutions that can make these tasks easier. Part 1 is designed to provide you with proven suggestions that can be and, in many cases, should be incorporated into your everyday life.

The information presented in Part 1 is designed to provide you with the ideas and electronic tools to "normalize" your life and provide you with more independence. Once you have implemented some of these recommendations, they can make your life easier. We understand that each of our needs is different, so we would suggest that you first turn to the chapter that is most important to you. And if you find the information in that chapter useful, we believe you are likely to find the other chapters just as helpful.

1

Creating Your Network

Aside from hermits, few of us go through our daily lives alone. Most of us have family, co-workers, neighbors, and doctors that we see and rely on. The problem is that when low vision occurs, the need to have other people help us with daily tasks increases greatly. The more severe the low vision is, the more important it becomes to have a network of trusted folks that you can count on to be there. If you have not done so already, putting together the names and contact information in an easy-to-access location, such as in a computer, in a smartphone, or on a sheet of paper, should be a high priority.

In this chapter, we will cover the most relevant groups of people and services that you should consider including in your network. You may already have someone there to help you, both in your home and in your community. You may be living with a spouse, partner, or relative who can help you with the tasks that you struggle with daily—to drive you to appointments, to visit friends and relatives, or just to get you out of the house for a while. Any one of them can help you put together your list of contacts.

For those others who may live on their own, it is equally important to reach out to someone you know and trust to help you create your "go-to" network, if you are unable to do it yourself. If you need help, just know that there are many services available to you. (See *Resources*, page 300.)

It is likely that your contact list will be based on several key factors—relationships, location, living space, costs, and personal and medical needs. Each of these factors will play a role in who you wish to include in your network. The following presents you with both the people and services to keep in mind as you put together your network.

YOUR SUPPORT TEAMS

Essentially, the people and services in your support group are there to help you deal with those responsibilities that you are no longer comfortable doing alone—or to provide you with the right technology in your home. Based on the relative severity of your low vision, these elements can include a wide range of tasks—from simply keeping you company to making sure that you get to your doctor's appointments on time. And even if you have a spouse or partner living with you, you need to make sure that the details of your support team—names, addresses, phone numbers, and emails, along with what services they may provide—are always kept in an easy-to-access location.

RELATIVES AND FRIENDS

Relatives who live nearby can be particularly helpful, especially if you have a trusting and close relationship. They can visit, take you out to eat with friends, do grocery shopping for you, and even aid you with your finances.

You may even turn to relatives who live at a distance for assistance. If they are good at money management and you feel comfortable with them, these family members could help you monitor your bank and credit card accounts for potential problems. And if you establish a joint checking account with them, they can write checks for you. They may even be able to order online items, like groceries or cleaning products, from a local store that can make home deliveries.

Some neighbors may also want to help, but they may not know how best to approach the topic with you. If you ask them, though, they—or their teenage children, if they have any—may be happy and willing to bring in your mail and packages, and may even agree to come into your home to sort out and open those things that you will need to use. They may be glad to mow your lawn in spring and summer, rake your leaves in autumn, or perhaps even shovel your snow in winter. They might even be willing to drive you to the store or to a scheduled appointment. It would be a thoughtful gesture to offer to pay a small sum of money to those helpful teens who may live in the neighborhood as a show of thanks for their time and effort.

As your vision issues continue to develop, you may want to ask a neighbor to keep their eye on your house to spot any potential problems, such as overflowing leaves in your gutters; a weakened tree that might be in danger of falling on your house; or any other potential damage to your house, roof, or yard that you may not be aware of. Addressing these problems at an early stage could very well prevent far more expensive repairs up ahead.

Good friends may also be willing to do some of these same tasks for you. They may pick you up for doctor appointments and arrange to have meals with you and other friends. They can take you to religious services or community events. You often do not know the extent of a friend's commitment and loyalty—until or unless you simply *ask*.

LOCAL UNIVERSITY STUDENTS

Many nearby colleges and universities can also serve as a good place to find someone to assist you. Most schools of this sort will post job offerings for their students on their websites. The first thing to do is to locate a school that is relatively close to your home. Once done, you can give the school a call to find out which department is in charge of such job postings. Each school seems to have their own way of providing this information to their students, so it would be best for you to reach out and find out how things work on their campus.

Once you contact the right department, you can ask how you can post your own particular job opening. In many cases, you will be asked to provide details about what the position entails. It would be a good idea to put together a general list of the tasks you would like the student to perform in advance.

In your posting you may state that the student must have access to a car. In addition, they would be responsible for going to a store, cleaning your house, taking your dog for a walk, preparing meals for you, cutting your grass, and so on. Obviously, you will know best what tasks you would like to have done.

Once you have hired and begun to work with a student in this way, you may go on to further develop a relationship with this person that can benefit you both. For example, you could work out an arrangement where you provide the student with room and board in exchange for their assistance as needed while they continue to attend classes. This could be a blessing for everyone involved.

TECHNICAL SUPPORT

It is likely that you may need assistance setting up technical devices such as those that we will be discussing in the coming chapters. If you do not have a knowledgeable partner, relative, or friend to help you, then your "next-door neighbor" teen may have all the skills required to be of service—and may even be delighted to help. However, in some cases, it will take a trained computer expert to properly install some of the devices that can make your life easier.

A nationwide organization for this kind of technical assistance is available from the "Geek Squad," which is associated with the popular *Best Buy* electronics stores. Those trained to be a "Geek Squad" representative are well-trained experts with the ability to set up, install, and repair different types of high-tech equipment and appliances. These include computers and tablets, smartphones, TVs, together with domestic home appliances like refrigerators, workout equipment, and others.

In addition, these individuals may have experience helping those with low vision like yourself—in particular, those who need *voice-activated* in-home tech products like Amazon's Alexa software and appliances like thermostats. The devices and appliances that the "Geek Squad" can install do *not* have to be purchased from *Best Buy* directly. To work with *Best Buy* technicians, however, you will need to invest in a *My Best Buy* total membership. (For more information, contact a *Best Buy* store nearest you.)

If you are not based near a *Best Buy* location, you can contact other nearby businesses that sell computer equipment—and ask if they offer that same kind of technical service. If they do not, you can ask them if they can provide you with the names and numbers of a few computer professionals who you can contact. You may wish to speak to several people to make sure you are getting the right person for your needs. It is also always a good idea to go onto the internet to read reviews of these stores and/or these computer professionals. When dealing with these companies or technicians, and *before* the start of a job, you should always ask for a *written* cost estimate and guarantee that they will repair their work for at least one year should their installed equipment not perform as was promised and/or advertised.

HOUSECLEANING

At a certain point, you may need someone to help you vacuum, dust, and clean your bathrooms and kitchen. Hiring the right person for this type of work is important. In order to keep your home clean, this person will normally have access to your entire house, so you want to hire someone who has a good track record for working hard and being honest. If you do not already have someone like that, ask friends and neighbors for a recommendation. They may be using a cleaning person they trust to do a good job.

If you are still not able to find someone to help, there are online cleaning services that you can contact and who will provide you with people to take care of your home. Whoever you select, it is important to make sure that your valuables are always stored in a secure location prior to their house cleaning visits. This applies to your financial records, as well.

And should the person you have entrusted to clean your home leave unexpectedly, it is a good idea to have a few other contact names in your network list.

FINANCIAL PERSONNEL

As mentioned earlier in this chapter, you will need people who are completely trustworthy and savvy with money to help you manage your finances. This might be a close relative, a trusted friend, an accountant, or even a professional financial advisor. The level of expertise you may need is likely to be based upon your income level. Still, you should always be aware of your personal finances.

Your bank and associated financial institutions should also have specially trained people who can assist you by granting you access to free "large-print" monthly statements and physical checks. They may also provide them in braille or in an audio format. (For much more on these kinds of details, see Chapter 9, *Your Money*, page 140.)

GROCERIES

If you do not yet have a good way to order groceries and have them delivered to your residence, there are several ways that you can have this done. As it turned out, with the pandemic lockdown came the advent of the "same day" food delivery services. Food shopping for many families using companies such as Amazon Fresh, Boxed, DoorDash, Instacart, Foodtown, Fresh-Direct, Hungryroot, Peapod, Shipt, Thrive Market, and Walmart became the norm. Today, most of these services have remained free of service charges, as long as a minimum dollar purchase is reached on each order. Each has their own minimum requirement, while others charge annual membership fees.

Here are a few key details regarding each of these different service providers:

■ **Walmart+ Plan.** If you have a Walmart+ Plan, then you can get groceries and other items delivered free from a local store within a day—and with no minimum amount. Walmart+ is a corporate membership program that combines in-store and online benefits to Walmart shoppers at an automatic yearly or monthly fee. Some credit card providers, like American Express, will cover the membership fee up to a certain amount. The *Walmart+ Assist Plan* is available to those who qualify for government assistance under the Supplemental Nutrition Assistance Program (SNAP), the Special Supplemental Nutrition Program for Women, Infants, and Children (WIC), Medicaid, and more. The Walmart+ fee is 50% less when receiving government assistance.

■ **Amazon Fresh.** Amazon Fresh is another service that delivers groceries to your door if you live in one of a number of large cities. Amazon Prime members may receive a discount off select grocery items. Just ask the voice-activated Amazon app called Alexa if this service is available in your city.

■ **Shipt, Instacart, and DoorDash.** These same-day delivery services work through your local grocery stores, pharmacies, restaurants—and even pet stores—to deliver to its customers a wide variety of items.

Because of the large number of delivery services available, take some time to find the one best suited to your own needs. It is also important to point out that all of these services use their own websites and/or apps for you to place your grocery orders. Because of this, you may need an appropriate computer screen device to place your orders. In addition, many of these services provide various other "perks" and additional services that may be of use to you—just be sure to explore all of your options.

HANDYMAN/HANDYWOMAN

Finding the right person who can do a variety of odd jobs around your house—both inside and outside—is important. From fixing simple plumbing, electrical, or appliance problems tor washing windows, painting walls or removing leaves from your home's gutter system, it is important to have a person or people in your network. If you do not have a reliable person to call on for any of these common problems, then ask your relatives, friends, and/or neighbors for some contacts. Of course, you may also need the names of plumbers, electricians, or painters based upon the level of work needed.

Always ask how much a potential job will cost before you allow any work to begin. In some cases, you may need a sighted person to oversee the work—just to make sure things are being done correctly.

MEDICAL PERSONNEL

It is very important to have a comprehensive list of your doctors and other healthcare providers—along with your pharmacy of choice—clearly identified and included in your network. In addition, you should list all the medications that you are on over time, including the dosage size of the meds and the suggested times that you should take them. Not only should you have this list legibly in-hand within your home, but this information should also be made accessible to those of your relatives, friends, and/or neighbors to whom you feel closest. It is important to find those people who will make an extra effort to help you address your health needs—while always keeping your low-vision challenges in mind.

As you probably are aware, medical emergencies can arise unexpectedly, so having this list handy is very important—and it should be kept up to date. Keep in mind that the doctors we see today may not be the doctors we will be seeing in the near-future. And while we have touched upon the importance of the medical information put into your list, the topic of healthcare will be discussed in more detail in Chapter 10, *Health Matters*.

PUTTING TOGETHER YOUR LIST

If you find yourself struggling to read your own personal lists of telephone numbers that you had written out "by hand" before the start of your vision problems, here is one way to solve the problem. Ask someone to make a list of your most commonly called numbers using a personal computer (PC) word processing software like Microsoft Word or some other similarly designed computer word program. Put the name of each contact on the left, and have the telephone number placed on the right. Under the name on the left, include some form of information identifying the name above. Skip a space and go to the next time.

Ask that this be done for you using a large-sized letter (font), so that you can see it more easily. Putting your entries into **boldface** may also help you to see them better. You may want to also underline the name and phone number of each entry, so you can easily find the right number for the right person.

Include names of relatives, friends, neighbors, local government and utilities, personal care individuals, medical offices and pharmacies, service people, and so on. Print these sheets out from a computer—if you do not have one yet in your home, you can ask the person who is helping you with this to save the file and print either from their own home printer or print it at a local library or a store like Staples. Buy an inexpensive three-ring notebook and several three-hole individual plastic folders, and slip one sheet each into its own separate folder—this will help protect each page from needless wear and tear. You can then organize these sheets in your notebook any way that makes sense to you. Now you have your own *personal* phone book.

There are three ways that you will need to make that assembled list available to you, as you will learn in the coming chapters. First, you can put it into your computer and print out the list in a large-size font. Second, you can write it down on a sheet of paper, so that you and other people can access your list. And third, you can have the information inputted into Amazon's voice-activated Alexa app to ask her for the phone numbers when you need any of them.

Keep all the written material you've gathered in one brightly colored folder that you can easily see.

The network you have now put together is there for many reasons. Having that list handy will definitely make your life easier. Whether it's having the names of people to call upon to perform a variety of skills or to simply have someone to reach out to for advice, that list will make a difference. It will take time to put it together, but it will be worth the effort—both now, and in the long run.

HOME PERSONAL ASSISTANT (HPA)

At a certain point, it may become necessary to have a full- or part-time person to help you with the various everyday tasks that need to be done—from cleaning your home to taking you out for a walk. This type of person is referred to as a Home Personal Assistant or HPA. There are also medical aides whose responsibilities are different from HPAs, because they have extra skills to provide medical attention but do not help you around your house.

When interviewing a person for such an assistant position, it is important to consider having a friend, relative, or neighbor with you. Learning about the person's background and being able to speak to others who the aide may have worked with is also a helpful step in the process. And while you may never need such a person, having a dependable contact in your network for such a person or agency will never be a bad thing to have.

Finding a HPA

There are a number of ways to locate a potential home personal assistant. There are in-home aide agencies that can be contacted or an ad can be placed online or in a local newspaper, or you can consider the following steps:

■ **Place of worship.** Ask your minister, rabbi, or imam if there is anyone in the congregation who would be interested in helping you part-time for a fee. If you need help 24/7, ask if there is someone who would be interested in living with you for free room and board in exchange for assisting you. Check this person out well and make sure you are both compatible.

■ **Care.com.** This company's website provides a wide variety of care providers, from pet care to housekeeping to senior care. You just enter your zip code and answer questions about the types of services you need, how soon, and how many hours. Pictures of possible candidates will pop up and you can click on them for more information. (See *Resources*, page 305.)

■ **Medicaid.** Another way to find an HPA for low-vision or blind persons is through Medicaid, provided that you are currently receiving benefits at the time of your inquiry. Medicaid offers a wide range of home services including personal care, homemaker services, and even relief for caregivers who are exhausted. The goal is to keep you in your own home—not only because it will be better for you, but because it will also be cheaper for the state than having you moved to a nursing home or some other similarly appointed outside institution. Care management is provided by a team composed of a nurse and social worker. To qualify, you must meet certain income and resource requirements.

Each state has different programs and eligibility rules. For more information, be sure to contact your state Medicaid office. (See *Resources*, page 307.)

Paying for Home Personal Assistants

If you cannot afford to pay for a Home Care Assistant, here are some ways to receive extra benefits for yourself—so that you can then have the available cash to do so.

■ **Health insurance policies.** Check your healthcare policy. Generally, companies don't offer long-term home services. However, some commercial insurance companies will pay for skilled professional home healthcare experts under a cost-sharing plan.

■ **Social Security benefits.** You may qualify for Social Security benefits if you have low vision or blindness. There are two programs to look into:

■ The **Social Security Disability Insurance (SSDI)** program and the **Supplemental Security Income (SSI)** program. To learn more about applying for assistance from either/both entities, you can call them or go on their website. (See *Resources*, page 310.)

■ **Veterans' benefits.** If you are a veteran with low vision or blindness, you may find the Veterans Administration (VA) helpful. Contact the Visual Impairment Services Team (VIST) at your nearest VA regional center. The VA offers rehabilitation and home modification services to help veterans live an independent life. These include orientation camp; mobility training, counseling, and providing needed assistive technology.

Home improvements and home modifications may be provided to make your home safer based upon your needs and how well you function with your visual loss. On the internet, be sure to also enter the partial phrase "VA blind and low vision rehabilitation services" into the Search window of whichever web browser you or a member of your support team may use when searching for things online. (See *Resources*, pages 303 and 311.)

Finding the right HPA could make all the difference when it comes to you being able to get help with those many tasks that you can no longer take on and complete for yourself. He or she could become a helpful trusted friend who makes your life better and so much easier—and also helps you stay safely in your home, which you have clearly come to love and treasure over the years.

CONCLUSION

Putting this information together will take some time and effort. In the end, though, you will find the effort well worth it. As you collect these names, keep in mind what expenses may be associated with some of these contacts. If you have the money to spend on updating your home and being able to equip your surroundings with all the latest gadgets and devices, then that is great.

If you have a limited budget, however, then just make sure your network reflects what you can afford. Your low-vision challenges do not necessarily need to have a high price tag attached to them. Just be sure that you have set up for yourself a system based on careful planning and the support of a team of people to whom you can turn for help—or even just a good laugh, which is something so many of us could use from time to time.

2

Virtual Assistants

Over the last few years, there has been a revolution in assistance technology for those with poor to no vision. With the development and use of machine learning (ML) and artificial intelligence (AI), a new world of help is now available for those who face visual challenges. In plain English, this technology allows computer programs to verbally answer questions that are asked, offer information, provide directions, take commands, and convert spoken words into text. This is truly a game changer.

Over the last few years, AI software has been incorporated into a number of devices. These devices can not only assist us in our everyday tasks—they can also open our worlds to so much more. As you will learn, these devices are available in two forms—those that are *mobile*, and those that are *stationary*. In this chapter, we will discuss the most commonly used devices that are available along with the AI programs that go by the names of Siri, Google, Bixby—and, of course, Alexa.

MOBILE DEVICES

Mobile devices provide their users the ability to travel outside of their homes. While the most common of these devices are smartphones, there are a few others to be aware of as well. Since it is likely that many of our readers may already have smartphones, it is important to make sure that we always take full advantage of these devices.

SMARTPHONES

Like our old cell phones, smartphones allow you to make and receive calls, emails, and texts—but with the use of new AI technology, they can perform these tasks through verbal instructions. You tell it what you want done, and as long as it falls within its wide range of functions, it will do it. Just as important, these smartphones can read out loud the words that appear on the screen and verbally identify apps for you to open—all on your command.

Choosing a Smartphone

There are several different types of smartphones available, all of which have similar features. However, many of the additional features are available at various prices. What follows are important features to look for if you have low vision.

WHAT CAN A SMARTPHONE DO FOR YOU?

Here are just a few of the things you can do using your spoken commands:

- Make phone calls by name.

- Track your location.

- Call "9-1-1" in case of an emergency.

- Search the web for information.

- Give you the time and weather.

- Provide the latest news and sports.

- Open an app.

- Read information on a screen.

- Increase the size of the copy on a screen.

- Read ebooks out loud.

- Play your favorite music.

- Get recipes and cooking instructions.

- Keep lists of needed groceries.

- Set a reminder to do something.

- Turn it into a magnifier.

■ A **large, clear, and bright screen** that has levels of contrast and magnification that can be set.

■ A **voice assistant** that helps you perform various everyday tasks. Alexa, Google, Siri, and Bixby are all examples of voice assistants that we will discuss later in this chapter.

■ A **screen reader** can read aloud to you everything that is on the screen, from your device's battery level to which app your finger is on. This feature can read texts, emails, and ebooks as well as the information available on most apps and websites.

■ A **"Talkback"** feature, which describes things you select on the device's screen, such as icons, buttons, or features. It works on every screen, even when you are browsing the web, sending text messages, or taking photos. It also provides suggestions for certain apps frequently used, and will help let you know what to do based on your past actions and usage patterns. Talkback is Google's built-in screen reader, and is available on any Android smartphone purchased today.

■ A **text-to-speech** feature, which both converts your speech to text and also reads text aloud to you. This feature is available on both Androids and iPhones today.

■ A **camera** that can take a picture of text, objects, faces, colors, and even barcodes, and describes them aloud to you.

■ A feature that allows you to **adjust the speaking rate and pitch** to suit your needs. *VoiceOver* is a built-in screen reader in iPhones and iPads.

■ A feature that uses your **fingerprint, sensor, or facial recognition** to unlock your phone without the use of a password.

If you are not a tech-savvy person, then it is important to find someone who is. Talk to your tech person about the special features you need, given your present level of sight. You can also go to the individual smartphone stores to ask questions to learn which model may be the easiest for you to operate and understand.

SMARTPHONE BRANDS

The most popular smartphone brands include Android, Galaxy, Google Pixel, Motorola, Samsung, and the Apple iPhone. They all come with a voice-activated feature and a screen-reader feature. All of these features need to have their settings turned on in order to work. All of them, except for the Apple iPhone, are based on the Google program.

NOTHING IS PERFECT—YET

When using a smartphone, there will be times you will run into a website that is not low-vision friendly. For example, when trying to arrange for a car ride, you may be required to put in a code texted to you to confirm your identity. You are then supposed to take that code and enter it into the space provided by the car ride's website. The problem is the code is too small to read, or the code is in the middle of sentences, making it impossible to have the smartphone read it back to you correctly.

Unfortunately, there may be a number of situations that leave you in a similar dead end. And as frustrating as that is, you will need to come up with alternatives to use when it does happen. For example, if the car services website doesn't allow you to locate a ride, make sure you have the phone number of a local taxi service available in your phone. If you plan to use the service of a specific website you have not used before, test it out prior to having to use it. If one thing doesn't work, you need to come up with one that does. Just remember to be prepared when it does happen.

Apple iPhone uses its own Siri program to operate these features. However, the Google program can be added to an iPhone, but Apple's Siri and Google programs cannot be used together. One must be turned off, while the other is turned on.

Android, Galaxy, Google Pixel, Motorola, Samsung

All of these smartphone brands have the following features built into their programs. To turn on these features, go to your "Settings" app, look for the appropriate setting, and slide the button to the "On" position.

■ **Voice-activated feature.** Once the setting has been turned on, by saying "Hey, Google" or "Okay, Google" to all but one of these models, you can speak into your phone to have it send texts, set reminders, read emails, make calls, and ask questions. You can open apps and select music. It can also allow you to control basic system settings. The Samsung smartphones, however, require you to say "Hi, Bixby" to activate all these features.

■ **Screen-reader feature.** "Talkback" can provide audible descriptions of what's on your screen—from texts and emails to your smartphone's battery level or who may be calling. You can also adjust the speaking rate and pitch to suit your needs.

■ **Additional benefits.** By having the Google program in your smartphone, you can use voice commands to control Google-programmed alarms, lights, thermostat controls, and much more in your home.

With Microsoft's free Seeing AI app on Android phones, you can set it up to recognize the people in your life, identify currency, read text, scan barcodes, and have a description of the scenery that is in front of you.

Apple iPhones

Apple iPhones have the following features built into their programs. To turn on these features, go to your "Settings" app, look for the appropriate setting and slide the button to the "On" position.

■ **Voice-activated feature.** By saying "Siri," you can speak into your iPhone to have it send texts, set reminders, read emails, make calls, and ask questions. You can open apps and select music. It can also allow you to control basic internal system settings.

■ **Screen-reader feature.** VoiceOver provides audible descriptions of what's on your screen—from battery level, to who's calling, to which app your finger is on. You can also adjust the speaking rate and pitch to suit your needs.

■ **Additional benefits.** By having the Google program in your iPhone, you can also use Microsoft's free Seeing AI app to identify currency, recognize people, read text, scan barcodes, and have a description of the scenery that is in front of you.

A CAUTION REGARDING SCREEN-READING PROGRAMS

Screen reading features for smartphones and computer devices work reasonably well when the text on the screen appears in sentence form as straightforward copy. A problem arises, however, when the copy that appears on the screen is a code such as "SQ12pG" or when the words are mixed with images. In most cases, the reading feature cannot decipher this type of copy correctly.

Here is an example: Since so many companies now send out a follow-up code to confirm it is you who has requested something to be done through their website, it is likely that the reading feature will not be able to verbally provide you with the code. By being aware of such issues beforehand, you may arrange to have someone with you to read these codes. Be aware that the reading feature is not yet perfect, and can sometimes be frustrating.

Apple also makes an Apple Watch that has many of the features of the Apple iPhone, except that it is smaller and worn around your wrist. It can operate with the iPhone close at hand, or for an extra monthly fee, it can operate without the iPhone being close at hand. However, in order for you to purchase an Apple Watch, you must show proof that you or a friend currently own an iPhone. And just like the iPhone, it provides both the command and screen reading features—which makes it more convenient to use once these features are turned on. However, keep in mind that its display screen is much smaller than the iPhone screen.

VIRTUAL REALITY HEADSETS (VR HEADSETS)

These headsets were initially developed for virtual reality gamers. Worn on the head, the game programs would be seen on the display in front of their eyes. The players could control their characters' actions by using a handheld control. As the headsets' technology improved, control could be done through eye movement, hand movement, and vocal commands. The same devices can now be used to assist persons with low vision. By adding specialized software into the headset, the following adaptive technology features are offered:

■ A **clear and bright screen** that has levels of contrast and magnification that can be permanently set or modified as needed to view text or photos.

■ A **screen reader** can read aloud to you everything that is on the display. This feature can read texts, emails, and ebooks as well as the information available on most apps and websites.

■ A **text-to-speech** feature, which both converts your speech to text and also reads text aloud to you.

■ A **camera** that can take a picture of text, objects, faces, and colors, which can then magnify the image taken.

■ A feature that allows you to **adjust the speaking rate and type of voice (male or female)**.

Wearing these headsets may not be for everyone. These issues will be covered in Chapter 13, *Magnification Options* (see page 233).

SMALL COMPUTER TABLETS

Another mobile device to consider is a small computer tablet. There are a number of companies that manufacture these tablets. They include Google, Samsung, and Amazon. As it turns out, nearly all these tablets can have the same features as a smartphone. Once your tablet is connected to the internet, you can add apps that will allow your tablet to listen to your commands, read screens, make calls, and more.

And unlike smartphones, you can select a much larger screen to view images and copy. In addition, most tablets—and computers—have a zoom setting that, when turned on, can enlarge the copy on the screen. (This feature is not connected to the widely used Zoom meeting program.)

If you have a tablet produced by Google, just like a Google-based smartphone, you can also set it up for you to use voice commands to activate Google-controlled alarms, lights, and thermostat controls, and much more in your home. With the Amazon tablet, you can do the same through use of Siri-controlled devices in your home.

THE "SMART" CANE

The long walking cane has been the traditional mobility aid used by those with severe vision loss or blindness. It simply allowed the person using it to alert themselves to potential obstacles in their path. Today, however, it can be added to the list of virtual assistants. The WeWALK handle attaches to any long cane, which turns the cane into an electronic mobility aid.

It was designed to feel natural, allowing for normal cane usage. However, when the user is walking, the cane will vibrate to indicate the presence of low-hanging obstacles that the bottom of a standard long cane may typically miss, such as a sign or tree branch. Users may also upload an app in their smartphone that will allow them to listen to information, which coordinates with the cane to assist them in finding their location and public transportation. (See Chapter 11, *Aids for Those Who Are Blind*, page 193 and *Resources*, page 323.)

STATIONARY DEVICES

A number of years ago, there was an invention that became available called the Clapper. Once installed on a lamp's wall plug, all you had to do was clap your hands and the lamp's light would go on. Clap your hands again, and the light would turn off. It helped folks avoid having to get up and walk over to the lamp and turn the lamp switch "On" or "Off." For those with low vision, that simple device made a big difference. With the advancement of technology, we now have vocally activated smart home devices that can be attached to a lot more than lighting fixtures.

By just giving a spoken command, you can turn on your TV and change the stations, reset the thermostat, lock and unlock the front door, open and close blinds, and so much more. Almost all the things in your home that need to be activated by flipping a switch, pressing a button, pulling a cord, or repositioning a setting can be done now by just asking for it aloud. With virtual assistance, if it can be hooked up to an electrical control, your stationary object can be operated hands-free.

All these smart home devices need to have a specific app to work within a central control hub, smartphone, computer, and/or tablet. They also require Wi-Fi—wireless digital networking technology—to work. The four top companies that offer these smart home devices are Amazon, Google, Apple, and Samsung.

ALEXA

Alexa is part of the Amazon group of products. The Alexa app can be used on its mobile devices. It is also used to run its central hub called Alexa Echo, which acts as both a speaker and a microphone. As a virtual assistant, once set up, it can answer questions, set reminders, play music, make calls, and set up personal emergency contacts. According to Amazon, it has over 90,000 functions. It can also be operated by an app on your smartphone, tablet, or computer.

To support Alexa, Amazon offers many entertainment- and security-based products. Alexa can also interface with a number of other manufacturers' smart home products, including both Google Nest and Apple HomeKit products.

GOOGLE NEST/GOOGLE HOME

Google provides the *Google Nest* app and *Google Home* app, which does not have the wide-range conversational features that Alexa has. Instead, these two apps work with its Google Nest Hub and mobile devices to allow the user the ability to use vocal commands that control all of its smart home devices. This includes cameras, speakers, locks, thermostats, Wi-Fi routers, and all Google Chromecast devices. These apps can be used on a smartphone, a tablet, and on a computer. The apps provide you the opportunity to verbally control all these devices. When set up correctly, they can also work with Alexa, as an added benefit.

APPLE HOMEKIT SERVICES

Apple offers the *Apple HomeKit Services*, also called *Apple Home*. It is similar to the Google Nest app in that it can control a wide range of smart home devices such as locks, door and window sensors, cameras, alarms, and motion detectors. The *Apple HomeKit* app provides you with Siri to verbally control your devices. It can be used on its hub, a smartphone, a tablet, and/or on a computer. It can also work with Alexa.

SAMSUNG (SMARTTHINGS)

Samsung offers the SmartThings app. It controls the SmartThings Hub. This is also similar to the Google

Home and Apple HomeKit Services app in that it provides control over a wide range of smart home devices such as kitchen appliances, door and window sensors, cameras, thermostats, and motion detectors. The app provides you with Bixby to verbally control your devices. It can be used on a smartphone, a tablet, and/or on a computer. And just like the Apple HomeKit, it can also work with Alexa.

SELECTING WHAT YOU NEED

In addition to the devices made specifically by Amazon, Google, Apple, and Samsung, there are many other companies that produce similar devices and appliances that work with these systems. However, and just as important, many of these products can work independently as well. They simply need a Wi-Fi connection to be linked to a smartphone, tablet, or computer. (See *Resources* section for company names, page 323.)

There are two important things to keep in mind when selecting an assistive system for your home. First, while all these companies' apps are free, their control center hubs and related devices and services that go along with them can be costly. So before selecting the system and/or devices that will work best for you, always ask how much this equipment and installation will cost, and if there are any monthly fees associated with some of their add-on services.

Second, before you purchase one of these assistive systems for your home, make sure to select smart devices and appliances that are all compatible with the system you are going to have installed. And if you find any of this is confusing, do not be afraid to ask questions. And if necessary, talk to someone who understands what needs to be done and can help you through the process.

There are a number of computer stores throughout the country that provide full services to set up such systems in your home, and to offer periodic maintenance if required. Before calling any of them, consider the kinds of *virtual* assistance you will need—now, and in the future. When you call, tell them what type of help you will need. Make sure you shop around, and just as important, read the reviews the store's service has gotten. And remember, you don't have to do everything at once. Additions to virtual assistance can be made over time.

ABOUT PRIVACY

You may be concerned about privacy issues when you use your smartphones and smart assistants. For instance, you may wonder if someone could listen to you and hear what is spoken. The unavoidable fact is that your smart assistant or smartphone is always eavesdropping. This is, and isn't, as creepy as it sounds. Although it is true that the device can hear everything you say within range of its microphones, it will normally first listen for its "wake up" word before it actually starts recording anything. For example, saying Alexa wakes up your Echo device from Amazon. Once it hears that word, everything in the following few seconds is perceived to be a command or a request and is swiftly sent up to Amazon's cloud computers, where the correct response is triggered *back*.

Of course, for those who have low vision or blindness, the advantages of these devices far outweigh the risks. As you know, these smart devices can improve the quality of your life in endless ways. Still, if privacy is a major concern, be aware that all listening devices can normally be turned off. All you need to do is know how it's done, and you can have the security you want whenever you need it.

CONCLUSION

If you lived a century ago—or even ten to twenty years ago—and had low vision or blindness, your life would have been considerably limited—no way to play music, read books, call friends, or summon help. But in today's world, smart devices are dramatically changing the way those with vision problems can live a much more normal life. Join the twenty-first century and enjoy its many technological miracles.

3

Safety Within Your Home

You may have lived in your house or apartment for many years, and over time, you have become very comfortable with your living arrangement. That is perfectly normal, however, problems may arise when your eyesight is weakened. Various sections in your home that you walk through every day may now become an "unseen" risk to your well-being.

In this chapter, we will offer several proven suggestions that may help decrease these risks and increase your safety. While many of these suggestions are not difficult or expensive to carry out, there are a few that may be somewhat costly. The important thing is to recognize what may need fixing to avoid any potential dangers in your home.

HOME SECURITY ISSUES

Safety may begin by having a secure home to live in—one that can protect you from burglars or unwanted intruders entering your home. Most of the following suggestions are designed for private homes.

FRONT DOOR LOCKS

Many people with low vision struggle to put a key in a lock. It can be very frustrating to try to find the right key, only to then try to get the key inserted into the door lock. While you might keep the appropriate key placed near the door, and feel your way to the key-hole, there are now a number of high-tech options available to deal with this problem. Again, it is important to point out that some of these methods can be expensive.

■ **Keyless entry door lock.** Today, all traditional key door locks in a home can be converted to keyless electronic locks. These locks can be opened or closed by adding a special app on your smartphone. You simply open the app and press a button on your phone. If you are unable to do that, but you have a voice-activated smartphone, just use a verbal command to lock or unlock the door.

Trustworthy people who need access to your home can put the same app on their smartphone and use the security code. The voice command can also be tied into your Alexa programs to allow you to lock or unlock the door on your command.

■ **Keypads.** An alternate consideration is installing a keypad-based lock. If you can see or feel the digits, then you can lock or unlock the door by pressing the correct numbers on the keypad. For such a lock, a keypad is placed on the outside door frame and in the home. If that is still a problem, the next method should work for you.

■ **Fingerprint locks.** Another high-tech method is to buy a special lock that uses your fingerprint. In the same way that smartphones can be opened by you putting a finger on the screen, this system allows you to lock the door from the outside when you leave home using a similar system. When you return, you again touch the lock with your finger, and the door unlocks. These units also use regular keys that you can give to those who may need entry into your home such as relatives, friends, or neighbors.

■ **Face recognition locks.** In the same way that millions of people have access to their smartphones through face recognition, the same technology can be used to unlock doors. By adding the photo device next to your door, the system can record the faces of all those you wish to have access into your home. It is important to have a device that incorporates a 3D depth program to make sure a photograph of a face cannot be used to unlock the door.

HOME ENTRY IN CASES OF EMERGENCY

What about in an emergency where police, firemen, or ambulance EMTs need to enter your home, but they don't have the key or password? This is important and easily solved. You can buy a special red box, universally recognized by emergency personnel, that look like the images below:

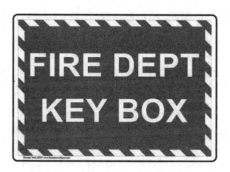
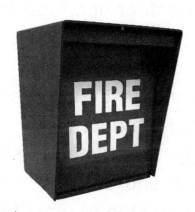

This kind of box is attached to your house in a prominent spot near your front door. Emergency workers throughout the U.S. know the universal code or have a key to open the box. Inside you keep a key to your front door. So instead of breaking a window or a door they can quickly enter to assist you.

In the box you can also include a sheet of paper that lists phone numbers of relatives and friends who should be notified, a list of our health problems, and a list of medications that you may currently take.

■ **Garage door opener.** If you have a garage attached to your home, there is a much less expensive option to consider. If your garage door is motorized and your garage has an inner door to your house, just keep the inner door in the garage unlocked. When you leave home, keep the front door locked, and leave through the garage. Simply carry the garage door opener in your purse or pocket, using it to open and close the garage door upon leaving or entering your home.

Just as your door lock can be opened by an app on your smartphone, for an additional expense, you can convert the garage door motor to one that responds to such an app.

You may want to stop by or call your nearest fire station and/or police station to make sure the red box that you plan to install will work on their end.

HOME SECURITY SYSTEM

Beyond locked doors and closed windows, there is the matter of home security system installation—one that triggers an alarm when set off, has a "24/7" monitoring service, and may even include recorded video. And should your alarm go off, it can automatically phone a relative or friend that there may be a problem at your residence. There are many such services from which you can choose. The costs of each system can vary widely, based upon the features you wish to include.

When shopping for a home security system, make sure to ask how the system can be turned on and off by someone who has low vision. Just like a fingerprint lock, they may have a similar device for people who cannot use a keypad. In addition, always have an alarm device to turn off or on as part of the alarm near your bed.

If you already have an alarm system set up in your home, you may want to have a fingerprint device added to your keypad system.

Ring Security System

One of the most high-tech security devices to become available was from a company now called Ring. It was the first to use Wi-Fi to detect movement and capture images of people at the front door of a home. Today, it has expanded to become a full-blown security system—one that can be tied into your Alexa program to take oral commands. And while it does require someone knowledgeable to install the system, it can be limited to the bare necessities of watching what goes on outside and inside your home—or it can come with an extensive amount of add-on services.

For someone with low vision, it will be difficult to see on a smartphone who is outside your door. However, the image can be hooked up to your television screen to view a large image—as long as your screen is tied into the Alexa program. In addition, even if you are not home, when your smartphone rings to let you know someone is at your door, you can talk to them through your phone, and they will hear you as though you are home.

A WORD OF CAUTION REGARDING THE INSTALLATION OF HIGH-TECH EQUIPMENT

Installing any high-tech security equipment is usually not cheap. You need to ask a lot of questions before-hand, such as: How long is the equipment guaranteed to work? Is there an additional service contract you will need once the guarantee period has passed? Who do you contact if the equipment doesn't work? Can the equipment be integrated into your existing home pro-grams, or do you have to buy an additional device or program to make it work correctly? While these devices are designed to help make your life easier, you don't want to discover that you have been taken advantage of in the process.

ELECTRICAL SHOCKS

Normally, all high-tech equipment is required to be plugged into electrical wall sockets. However, it's important to keep in mind that inserting plugs into outlets can be frustrating and potentially *dangerous*. If you cannot see the prongs of the cord and the insertion holes properly, you will fumble and could shock yourself if you touch the live smaller prongs incorrectly or plug them in the wrong way.

■ **Smart plugs**. Smart plugs from Amazon respond directly to Alexa commands. Ask someone to help you follow the easy instructions: you insert the smart plug into an outlet, and give it a name you'll remember such as "Plug 1" using Alexa. You can then turn it on by saying, "Alexa, turn on Plug 1" or "Alexa, turn off Plug 1." This is an easy, inexpensive way to solve a potentially dangerous problem.

PREVENTING FALLS

Falls are common in the home, especially among seniors with physical limitations and/or low vision. The riskiest places are stairs, the bathroom, and the kitchen. There are a number of simple things you can do to avoid accidental falls.

OVERHEAD LIGHTING

A common factor with many falls is poor lighting. Where once it was easy to avoid tripping over the edge of a rug or hitting the corner of a low table, today, it's a lot less easy to spot. Keeping all areas well-lit with bright overhead lights will help you see obstacles that might be in your way. Smart light bulbs can also be turned on by a voice command to Alexa. There are also light bulbs that turn on by clapping your hands.

STAIRS

Unfortunately, falling down a staircase can cause a great deal of bodily harm. Every staircase in your house should have a sturdy handrail that you can easily grip. There are a number of safeguards to keep in mind.

■ **Non-slip surfaces.** The stairs should have non-slippery surfaces. If you have a carpet going down your staircase, consider replacing it with anti-slip treads. It may not be as pretty, but it will be a lot safer.

■ **Count your steps and/or use a long cane.** You may need to keep track in your mind how many steps there are in a particular staircase. Count them so you don't miss a step or take an extra step at the bottom, causing you to fall. If you have been taught how to use a long cane when descending stairs, the cane will detect the last step down.

■ **Keep the stairs clear of objects.** People tend to leave objects on the bottom of staircases that they intend to bring up later. Unfortunately, a person going down those stairs can easily trip over those items. If you have grandchildren, make sure they have not left any toys on the stairs after a visit.

■ **Avoid using dangerous stairs**. Some staircases can have short step footings or are pitched at an extreme angle. They may also have a poorly placed railing. If you have a staircase like that in your basement, avoid using them. Instead, ask someone to retrieve what you need. If you have no other choice, add a non-slip surface to each step—and again, make sure the hand-rail is sturdy and in the appropriate position.

Options

If going up and down the stairs becomes a problem, consider a riding staircase in which you sit on a chair that takes you up or down stairs. This definitely avoids keeping you from falling down the stairs if you have physical and visual difficulties.

Another consideration is to move to a home with no staircases, where all the rooms are situated on one level. It is not always easy to leave a home you have lived in for years. However, it is a way many people choose to go to avoid the stress of worrying about falling down the stairs.

If you have balance problems due to your vision or other physical reasons that make you fall, ask your doctor for a referral to physical therapy. In only a few sessions, these therapists can teach you ways to improve your balance and give you balance exercises to do at home.

BATHROOMS

Your bathroom is potentially the most dangerous place in your home for falls. Bathroom floors made of slick tiles or linoleum and fiberglass or ceramic on the bottoms of your tub/shower can be very slippery when wet and soapy. Consider installing non-slip floors and use paste-on plastic safety strips in tubs and showers.

In addition, have a handyman install grab bars or place a plastic chair in your shower so you can sit down. Use bathmats outside the tub/shower cautiously because they can be easy to trip over.

If you enjoy taking a bath, but are afraid of slipping as you get out of the tub, you might consider replacing it with a walk-in tub. These tubs have a low entry step, non-slippery floors, and a built-in seat to sit down on while you fill the tub and enjoy the warm water. You might also get a showerhead that you can hold in your hand and position to wash your body, and maybe your hair.

If your balance is off, you may need someone to help you when you bathe. They can help you get in and out, hand you a towel to dry off, and then hand you clean clothes.

LOW-LYING OBJECTS

Reduce as much clutter on your floors as possible. Take control of your home environment. Put things away such as shoes, handbags, step stools, magazines, and so on—things that would be hard to see if you have low vision. Even pets can be a tripping hazard if their fur color is similar to the floor. Putting a contrasting- colored collar, a flashing light collar, or even bells on your pet may help alert you to their presence.

FURNITURE

In many homes, rooms are filled with a variety of items including tables, chairs, lamps, and vases. In order to navigate the room properly, you must walk around these objects. In the past, it was never a problem. However, with poor sight, bumping into or falling over one of these objects becomes a reality.

To avoid this problem, consider moving these pieces around each room to create straighter paths. If you cannot do it yourself, ask a relative or friend to help. While the room might not have the same pizzazz it once had, it will be a heck of a lot safer.

CONCLUSION

In this chapter you learned how to safe-proof your home. Ask someone close to you who knows your vision limits to go through your house with you in search of possible hazards, so that they can be corrected or eliminated.

On the other hand, as safe as your house might be, there is always the possibility of an unforeseen incident occurring in or outside your home. In the next chapter, we will address safety measures to deal with emergency situations.

4

In Cases of Emergency

Finding yourself in an unexpected emergency can be very upsetting. Creating a safe environment in your home is very important, but an unexpected injury or fall can happen anytime and anywhere. If anything happens that puts you in danger, the question you have to be able to answer is this: Do you have a way to reach out for help? Today, there are a number of high-tech devices you can use to ensure that you get help immediately. In this chapter, we will focus on the latest and most convenient devices that will help you to access these emergency services.

EMERGENCY SITUATIONS

Home emergencies can arise quickly and unexpectedly, putting you and a loved one in danger. They can also come in many forms—from a serious health issue to a home break-in. By anticipating the most common issues and preparing for them in advance, you can avoid any unwanted surprises.

CALLING 9-1-1 ON YOUR
LANDLINE OR SMARTPHONE

If you have an emergency, just dial 9-1-1 on your landline phone or smartphone. You can also use a voice-activated smartphone that will put through the call for you. Many smartphones have emergency dial features built in to contact police.

Each smartphone company normally comes with its own emergency contact system. It may be pressing and holding a side button that brings up the words "Emergency SOS" on the screen of an Apple iPhone. Or, it can be a verb command, such as "Hey, Bixby, call 9-1-1" on a Samsung Galaxy or "Hey, Siri, call 9-1-1" on an Apple iPhone, that helps you to call for help.

You should make it a point to learn what the features on your specific smartphone are to automatically dial for help. And remember to ask if your phone has the ability to track your location to get the help you need. While this feature is available in most smartphones, this feature must be turned on within your phone's settings in order to work.

Be Aware of Dead Ends

At this point, Alexa is not able to call 9-1-1 for you. However, you could tell her to call a friend who can then dial 9-1-1 for you. Or you could include in your

"Contact" list a non-emergency number for your local police, who could then immediately transfer you to 9-1-1.

THE APPLE WATCH

While the Apple Watch screen may be difficult to view for most people with low vision, its high-tech features make it a valuable device to have in case of emergency. To begin with, if you've taken a fall or been in a car crash, it will verbally ask if you've fallen or been in a crash. If you do not respond to the question, it will automatically call a designated emergency number for help. It will also provide your current location.

Additionally, in cases of a health issue, a fire, or a break-in, you can verbally request that the "Emergency SOS" icon appear, and ask it to call for help. Again, it will provide your location to that emergency service. You can also have several additional emergency contacts entered into its program, in case you need to call a relative and/or friend as well.

While an Apple Watch does not necessarily need an accompanying iPhone to work, it does require an iPhone for it to first be set up. This can be done using another family member's iPhone. After that is done, the only times that the same borrowed iPhone will need to be in range of your Apple Watch is for any mandatory software updates and tweaks that serve to update its settings. Also, be aware that there is an additional billing charge to have your Apple Watch work independently of an iPhone.

MEDICAL ALERT DEVICES

What if you are unable to call for help on any phone? In that case, you could wear a Medical Alert device that automatically connects you to 9-1-1, which can then send police, firemen, EMTs, or an ambulance to check on you. This is especially important if you live alone, or if your partner is often away from home. Also, if you fall in the shower or down some steps, you may likely not have access to your smartphone. A medical alert button, however, can always be present—as long as you remember to always wear it!

Some devices have no monthly fee while others do, which is paid automatically each month on your credit card. The company may supply a free monitor that is hooked to your landline. They also send you a button to be worn around your neck or a watch-like device worn on your wrist. These are waterproof and should always be worn, even in the bath or shower, because you never know when you might suddenly have an emergency.

There are a number of different medical alert devices available. The cost and services provided will vary. These are things to consider: Do you need a device for just your house and its immediate area, or do you need one that can also work when you are at a distance from home? Does it detect and report a fall that may knock you unconscious? Do you pay for the device upfront plus a monthly fee, or is it just a monthly fee? Are you asked regularly by the company to make sure your device is working?

Ask someone to go online for you and search for the "best medical alert systems." Or you could also discuss your options with your pharmacist, who may be able to show you several devices and advise you based on your needs and the price. (See *Resources*, page 335.)

FIRES/CARBON MONOXIDE DETECTORS

Whether you live in your own home or an apartment, your living facility should have both a fire and carbon monoxide detector. Make sure your smoke detectors have fresh batteries and are in working condition. Ask someone to test them every few months because if a battery is low and alerts you with an annoying "beep-beep" sound, you may not be able to fix it yourself.

If you smoke, you are at risk of easily starting a fire from a hot ember in your cigarette's ash that you may not see. Also, watch items you are cooking in the kitchen to make sure they don't catch fire as well.

HOME INVASIONS

Keep all doors and windows locked so that intruders will not have easy access to your home. Keep your garage door down and locked. You may want to keep lights on at night in a room or two, just to make it look like someone is home. If someone enters your home and presents a danger, you can quickly press your Medic alert button to summon help.

With homes that have a burglar alarm system, there is usually a button or two that will set off the alarm when pressed. Just the loud sound of the alarm going off should be enough to frighten them off. You may consider installing a security system to give you protection and peace of mind. Just keep in mind, when installing an alarm system, make sure it provides you with an easy way to be turned on and turned off.

MEDICAL ISSUES

Maintain a close relationship with your doctor or other healthcare provider to stay as healthy as possible. If you have major health problems, be sure you are following your doctor's instructions to prevent emergencies. Report any reactions to prescribed medications that make you sleepy or unsteady and more likely to fall. Discuss with your doctor or pharmacist your medications and any side effects.

CONCLUSION

In some cases, the suggestions in this chapter can be done by you alone. In other cases, you may need some help from a trusted relative, friends, neighbor, or any home care assistant, which should give you more peace of mind and help reduce your anxiety if you live alone.

Keep in mind that you may not only be paying for the device itself, but you may also be paying a monthly fee for the service. We suggest that you comparison shop to get the best price. You might also ask if there is a "disabled persons" discount available.

Hopefully, you may never find yourself in need of any emergency services. However, there is no reason to leave things to chance. The motto of the Boy Scouts is "Be Prepared." That is good advice to follow.

5

Living Well at Home

Our home lives are very important to each of us. It's where we carry out most of our daily routines. Whether it's work, entertainment, maintenance, or just relaxing, home is where we begin and end our day. And as time goes by, we take all these daily activities that we do there for granted. That is, until our sight begins to decline. The simple things that we did now become a lot more difficult. Well, at least that was how it was in the past, but now things have changed greatly. With the high-tech revolution marching forward, we now live in far better times.

As we have discussed in Chapter 2 on *Virtual Assistants*, with the advent of smartphones, Alexa, and other electronic devices, we now have the opportunity to get past many of the drawbacks that come with low vision. This does not mean that there won't be moments of frustration. The truth is that there will be challenges thrown your way that even these devices will not help you overcome. But, as you will learn in this chapter, there are many things you can do to regain control over your home, and to live a more normal life, even with low vision.

Before we begin, however, there is one very useful and relatively inexpensive tool you should always have within your reach—the magnifying glass.

A SIMPLE, BUT IMPORTANT TOOL

The magnifying glass comes in many forms and sizes, and it can become a quick tool to use for many purposes. In Chapter 13 on *Magnification Options*, you will find a variety of these to choose from based on the magnification you need, and the amount of light required. By having this tool nearby, you can read printed words that you might not otherwise be able to make out. Of course, you can also use a smartphone as a magnifier when you open its magnification setting, but you will find that a handheld magnifier with a built-in light works a lot quicker. It's just a matter of using it when you simply need it.

MAKING CALLS

While you may never have had a problem calling others, low vision can impact your ability to make phone calls or send out texts. It is likely that using landlines and cell phones as well as looking at your own personal list of phone numbers may become a frustrating experience. Today, however, there are a number of devices that can make calling easier. Let's start with the cheapest:

LARGE-PRINT LANDLINE PHONES

The numbers on a typical landline phone are printed small. You can use a magnifier, of course, but there are other options. Landline phones are available with large-print numbers displayed as shown below. Many phones can also be programmed to call specific phone numbers. With this particular model, you put the faces

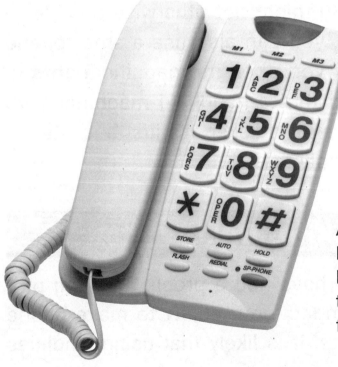

An easy-to-see big button telephone can be very helpful when trying to reach family, friends, and doctors.

of the people that you call often, so all you do is press the button covered by a photo of the person that you wish to call.

There are also many phone devices, such as an answering machine, that will announce who is calling you by the caller's phone number or by their name. If you do miss a call, most major phone networks will allow you to redial a missed call by dialing * 6-9, that is, star-six-nine.

SMARTPHONES

Most smartphones have settings to enlarge the size of the print that appears on their screens. You can also set the device to **BOLD** the text. Larger, bolder letters may help you see your contacts list to call numbers and to text.

If you still struggle to see on your smartphone screen, you could buy one that has a screen that folds open, so you have a larger screen with larger print options. For example, the Galaxy is a smart Android phone that folds open.

If you still struggle to see the text on a Galaxy or on other similar smartphones, then you can ask someone you trust to go to your phone's settings and activate the magnification setting. This will allow a magnifier to appear over the text which you can enlarge even more.

Voice-activated Smartphones

If you still cannot make out what's on the screen of your smartphone, you can go to the smartphone's settings and turn on the feature that makes your phone respond to voice commands. This lets you just ask your device to call your friend "Jane Doe" for you. You can also text messages to "Jane Doe" as well. You can order a carsharing service, purchase groceries, or confirm a doctor's appointment by just using your voice. You can also turn on the "Screen Reader" or "Talkback" setting to have your phone read aloud what appears on your screen.

MAKING CALLS THROUGH OTHER DEVICES

Just like voice-activated smartphones, you can ask your tech-savvy person to put your contacts list from your phone onto a computer, tablet, or device such as Alexa. Then all you have to do is say, "Please call 'Jane Doe' "—and it does!

There you have it. Current technology now provides many different ways to stay in contact with friends, family, and the outside world—from using simple, inexpensive devices that you already have to more expensive ones that use the miracles of cutting-edge technology.

TELLING TIME, SETTING ALARMS, AND REMINDERS

Knowing the correct time is vital for everyday living. Whether it's setting a specific time to wake up or to get to an appointment, we all need reminders on which we can rely. Here are some helpful devices:

Telling Time

Large-Print Clocks are available online and from the catalogs. (See *Resources*, page 335.) Clock faces come with white numbers on a black background or black numbers on a white background. Decide which clock face you can read better prior to purchase. This can make a big difference for some people with low vision.

Large-Print and Talking Watches

Look online for watches that have numbers large enough for you to see. They too are available with black numbers on white faces or white

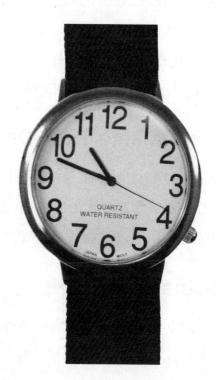

A large-print wristwatch can help with independence. There are also many wristwatches that speak the time and date.

on black faces, and that can make a difference for you. There are many versions from which to choose.

If you have trouble seeing your watch in low light, you may want a watch that also tells you the time out loud. You just press a button on the side, and you are told the time. Atomic watches, also called radio controlled watches, reset themselves each day receiving radio signals from a transmitter in sync to an atomic clock. They keep highly accurate time. A number of them come with electronic display screens that provide a large image of the time that you will be able to see more easily.

Most watches are available with the choice of two different wristband choices. One is a metallic expansion band that is easy to slip on. The second is a leather-type band, which may be harder to put on because of the little prong that needs to be put into a small hole. The choice of wristband should be simple.

Other Talking Time Devices

Voice-activated smartphones, the Apple Watch, and voice-activated assistants like Alexa will tell you the time and the date when asked.

Alarms and Timers

To wake you in the morning, you may need an alarm. Or in your kitchen (and elsewhere) you will often need to set timers. While you can always set times manually on your smartphone, by turning on the right setting, you can talk to your smartphone to set the time that you need for the alarm to go off. Or you can use a voice-activated assistant like Alexa to set a time for you. Just say, "Alexa, set a timer for 20 minutes." In 20 minutes, Alexa will tell you that 20 minutes have passed. Likewise, you can set an alarm. "Alexa, set an alarm for 7:00 am tomorrow."

Reminders

You can also set a reminder on voice-activated devices. "Alexa, remind me to take the garbage out every Wednesday afternoon at 5:00 pm." Or, "Alexa, remind me that I have a dental appointment at 1:00 pm on March 1st."

CLEANING THE FLOORS

Vacuuming or mopping up areas of the floor was never an issue in the past, however, with low vision, it can be. If cleaning the floors in your home becomes a difficult task, and you have no one to help you, there are self-propelled vacuums that can not only suck in the dirt but can mop the floors and carpets as well— all done hands-free. These machines set their own courses throughout your home. Each has an internal sensor, which allows it to safely navigate a path around the furniture and those stray objects on the floor. Once finished, it will return to a charging dock where it can then be recharged.

Best of all, it can be programmed to take voice commands through a smartphone, tablet, computer, and/or Alexa. iRobot Roomba offers a series of vacuums that work in this manner. These machines range in price based upon the features they offer. There are also a number of other similar self-operating vacuums to consider. It is therefore important to ask what features are available on any models that may work best for your home. They are relatively easy to install, but you may need a tech person to set up the voice control.

As for costs, consider this. Some of these machines can be pricey. However, over time, this expense could save you money compared to the cost of paying someone else to come to your home to vacuum.

With poor vision, should you be concerned about tripping over the machine once it's in operation? Normally, the sound of the motor will alert you to where the vacuum is working. However, to play it safe, have the machine work at a time when you are not roaming around your home.

COLOR FOR EASE AND SAFETY

When your eyesight is weakened it may be hard to see low-lying objects on the floor, such as the edges of cabinets or the handles on some doors. By using contrasting color tape, you can avoid unexpected falls or the frustration of trying unsuccessfully to open a cupboard or closet.

So, what *are* contrasting colors? Contrasting colors refer to bright colors that stand out when placed in front of a surface with a color that is less bright. For example, one can use a white tape placed against the edge of a black or similarly dark background. That white tape will now stand out. Of course, the color of that tape can be any number of colors as long as it stands out. Let's consider the following:

■ Bright colors are generally the easiest to see because they reflect light. So colors like red, orange, and yellow are more visible than pastels or pale colors.

■ Lighting can significantly affect your perception of color. You may have noticed that in dim light, colors may seem paler or "washed out," while bright colors appear more vivid.

■ Some colors may be difficult to distinguish when grouped with other similar colors—navy, blue, brown, and black; blue, green, and purple; pink, yellow, and pale green. These are the areas that need to be marked by a contrasting color.

■ Mark cabinets and edges of doors with brightly colored fluorescent tape. Or, apply a tape that has a rough surface that you can feel, which may also be helpful when locating handles and edges.

■ Use fluorescent or bright colored paint or tape to mark chairs, desks, steps, drop-offs, or workspaces.

■ Brightly colored chair cushions will help you see the chair better.

■ If your favorite chair is a dark color, drape a towel or Afghan in a contrasting color over the back of it.

■ A dark chair will stand out better if placed against a white or cream-colored wall.

■ Choose solid colors as background and avoid patterns, prints, or stripes. Some people prefer dark backgrounds while others prefer lighter-colored backgrounds.

■ Clear glasses and dishes are more difficult to see than colored ones, which makes it more likely that you may drop them or knock them off a table.

■ Carefully choose floor coverings—carpet, tile, or linoleum—so they provide a contrast to the wall colors. Also avoid carpets with patterns, especially on stairs. Placing white tape on dark steps or slopes may help you remember that there are more stairs ahead.

■ Wrap a contrasting color tape around door handles or on the edges of a cabinet mirror door to make them stand out better.

Keep in mind that these additions will likely require trial and error to determine what contrast works the best for you. Will these new colorful additions make your home more fashionable? Probably not. However, they *will* make your home safer, which in turn will make it easier to do the things you need to do with less stress.

WORKING IN YOUR KITCHEN

If you have been the one in charge of preparing meals, low vision can definitely make things a lot harder on you to carry out these duties. You will need to figure out the easiest ways to use your kitchen given your low-vision limits.

Again, let's start with simple devices and work up to the more complex, and likely, expensive ones.

ARRANGING YOUR KITCHEN

Low vision can make cooking rather difficult. It there-fore becomes important to know where everything is, or at least to have the ability to identify the locations of your cooking utensils and food. You can certainly do it yourself—but if you can't at this point, don't be embarrassed to ask someone to help you arrange your kitchen, so you can find things more easily. Take some time to think about how you want your drawers, cab-inets, and shelves organized, so it's easy to put your hands on what you need.

Going Back to Basics

Over the years, we tend to collect a lot of pots, pans, dishes, and other cooking utensils that we no longer use. The same thing is true with some of the food and staple ingredients that we keep in the pantry that we will either never use or that have gone past their expi-ration dates. Things that clutter up the kitchen. You should consider giving them away—or throwing them out. In other words, simplify your kitchen so you can find what you need more easily.

SHOPPING FROM HOME

Home delivery has improved immensely, especially with the advent of big companies like Amazon and Walmart. The pandemic has greatly influenced home delivery service as well. Having groceries and dinners delivered to your doorstep is very common these days and that is good news for persons who cannot get out on their own anytime they want. Shopping online or by using your smartphone can be quite convenient. Some stores you can just call, order your items, and ask that they deliver it. Other stores you can order online and they will deliver for a fee or free. For example, Walmart + customers can order online and have items delivered the same day free. Similarly, Amazon Fresh is an online grocery store but is not available in every zip code.

Many communities have delivery services like Shipt, Instacart, and DoorDash where you can order online from several stores, restaurants, and pharmacies. Having meals, medications, and groceries delivered to your door is a game changer for so many.

Location, Location, Location

When someone brings in groceries from outside your home, have them put those items that require refriger- ation or storage in your freezer in the same places— every time. Follow the same steps when it comes to your dry goods and/or cleaning solutions. All of these items should have their own established places on your counter, shelves, or cupboards. As you will dis- cover, it will save you a good bit of time having to hunt things down if things are always in the same location.

Label When Necessary

Many dry good packaging and containers look alike. Sometimes their labels can be hard to identify. If you are looking for cinnamon, you definitely do not want to inadvertently pick up the cumin powder. With pack- aged products that can be easily confused, take a magic marker and write down the name of the product on the packaging in large letters. And if the product name is too long to fit on the packaging, use a short- ened version that you can quickly recognize.

If it's still hard to identify the product, even after writing on it with a magic marker, place white tape on the product and write the name on the tape. It should now stand out.

Kitchen Appliances

If you struggle to see settings on various appliances like your microwave, stove, dishwasher, toaster, coffeemaker, and so on, you can use your handheld lighted magnifying glass as an aid.

If you still can't make out the settings, there are stick-on red dots that are sold that you can use to help identify some of the settings on your kitchen appliances. For example, on your stove, you can put a red dot on those temperatures you use most often, such as on the 350°, 400°, and Broil settings. On your dishwasher, place those red dots on the settings you use every day.

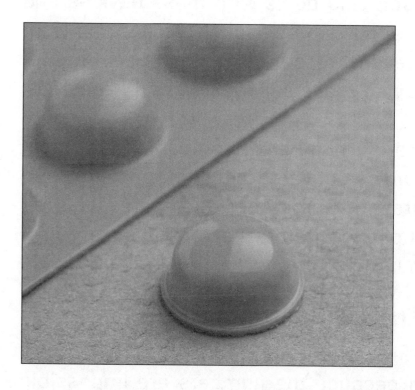

These high-contrast orange bump dots are great for marking buttons, keys on computer keyboards, and favorite settings on appliances and

Voice-activated Kitchen Appliances

Many different voice-activated kitchen appliances are now available. Of course, they must be paired with the right voice-activated devices like Amazon's Alexa or Google. There are microwaves, hot plates, coffee makers, and other small appliances. There are even large appliances like refrigerators and stoves that are now voice-activated.

Samsung makes these appliances, but they must be paired with either a Samsung smartphone or Alexa. Beware, though! These are much more expensive than their non-voice-activated counterparts because of all the technology involved. Get advice from a professional tech person who deals with these devices and can advise you about smart appliances and the right smart device needed to control them. (See Chapter 16, *Assistive Home Products*, page 271 and *Resources*, page 323.)

Today there are a number of companies that manufacture these voice-activated kitchen appliances, so always shop around. Sometimes there are sales on these smart appliance items that could save you a significant amount of money.

KITCHEN UTENSILS

Many kitchen devices do not work well for someone with low vision because the numbers are impossible

TAKING A BREAK FROM COOKING

Every so often, you might consider ordering in food from a local eatery. If it's within your budget, it can be done easy enough with one phone call. However, there are a few things to keep in mind. The first is selecting the food you wish to order. Normally, restaurants post their menus and prices on the internet. By going online and bringing up the menu on your smartphone, tablet, or computer screen and enlarging it, you can more easily see and make your take-out selections.

Once done, you call the restaurant to place your order for delivery to your home. Some local restaurants have their own delivery service to drop off the food. However, if the restaurant does not deliver food or it is too far away, you can have it delivered by Uber Eats, Lyft, Grubhub, or DoorDash among others.

These delivery companies charge an additional fee for their service. If you pay by a credit or debit card, you will be told what the cost is. If you plan to pay in cash, don't be shy about asking what the total cost would be prior to getting the food.

If you live alone, then you may want to ask a friend, neighbor, or relative over to your home to share a meal. It's a nice way to spend an evening.

to read. You could use red dots to mark most commonly used measures, but that is problematic if the device must be washed.

There are now other useful kitchen utensils to help in the preparation of a meal. For example, there are measuring cups and measuring spoons with extra-large or raised numbers you may be able to feel to identify the number. There are also talking food scales and measuring jugs. Special scissors will help you slice meats and vegetables without the use of a sharp knife. There are even smart meat thermometers that report to your smartphone the temperature of your meat as it cooks. (See Chapter 16, *Assistive Home Products*, page 271 and *Resources*, page 335.)

LAUNDRY

Washers and dryers typically have settings with small letters and numbers so when you need to purchase a new one, consider how easy to read the settings are.

Again, red dots can help. For example, on your washer you could place a dot on the temperature you use most often, the size of the wash, and the cycle length. You could do the same on your dryer. Put a red dot on the temperature you want and the time needed to dry.

Voice-activated Washer and Dryers

Just like voice-activated kitchen appliances, there are washers and dryers that can be controlled by voice commands. These machines can be controlled remotely by using a smartphone, a tablet, or talking to Alexa. These products are also pricey so it's important to learn as much as you can about these products, and always remember to shop around.

Many of the non-voice-activated suggestions can be done with a friend's help—all low-tech and very affordable. When considering voice-activated equipment, it is very important to work with professionals who know how to install and set up the equipment correctly. Initially, you may need a plumber to install the equipment in your kitchen and/or laundry room, and then you will need a computer tech to hook up the voice command to a smartphone, tablet, or Alexa. Make sure to ask for a warranty from the manufacturer, from the plumber, and/or from the tech prior to their installation of the product.

ASSISTED LIVING

This chapter has focused on the many things that are available to help you stay comfortably in your home where, hopefully, you would be the happiest. But we would be remiss if we didn't say that might not be the right solution for everyone.

There certainly are people with low vision who could benefit greatly by living in an assisted-living or senior care facility. There you would have people to help you in whatever ways you need assistance. This includes getting dressed, eating meals, getting medications on time, visiting with other residents, transportation to doctor appointments, perhaps grooming at a beauty salon and barber, a nurse and visiting doctor, and social activities. The decision to make such a change is not always easy.

Think it over, talk with close relatives, and visit a few facilities to see if one feels right to you. Prices vary considerably from place to place, and there may be organizations that may be able to help you financially. (See *Resources*, page 300.) Moving from where you have lived for years is never easy, but "home" is where you should feel happy, safe, and at peace.

CONCLUSION

As you may have come to understand, low vision can be very disruptive when it comes to doing the things you have done at home for years. It will take some time to adjust to many of these changes. However, as you have learned, there are many things you can do to make living at home more comfortable for yourself. In some cases, the changes are relatively easy to make. In other cases, the changes require that new devices be installed in your home.

Not everyone can afford a complete home make-over to make these changes. If money is an issue, the first thing you can do is make the changes that will cost you nothing or, at least, very little. Then consider what are the most important things you would like to have done that will cost money. Price out the devices, and learn how much you will be charged for having the equipment installed by a plumber, electrician, and/or a tech person. Remember that you don't have to buy everything at once.

If you take your time, you can comparison shop for both the quality of items and prices. Many devices do go on sale, so you can save a good deal of money by just waiting for the right time. If you find that this may be a little overwhelming, ask a friend or relative to help you through this process.

The suggestions in this chapter are all designed to make your home life easier. However, it is up to you to take the first steps. Simply put, low vision should not stop you from taking care of your home or yourself. In the next chapter, we will discuss the many things that can add some needed enjoyment to your life.

6

Entertainment

Having fun is important for everyone. It benefits each of us, both physically and mentally. Fun reduces our stress levels, boosts our mood, enhances our learning ability, improves our sleep, and so much more. And just because you have low vision, it should not be made an excuse for not enjoying your life. This chapter will help you choose the devices and fun activities that you can continue to enjoy, in spite of your vision issues.

In most cases, you will find the costs are minimal. All you need is a smartphone, tablet, computer, or Amazon's voice-activated Alexa software. Whether it's for amusement, education, or the mere pleasure of playing games, you will discover that you have many options to choose from—all of which may help to put a smile on your face. As you will learn, technology has truly opened a new world of entertainment. Let's begin by taking a look at one of the most common sources of entertainment in your home—your television.

LARGE SCREEN TELEVISION

Watching television can be entertaining, informative, and it can help expand your world beyond your home. However, watching TV on a small screen can be extremely frustrating if you have low vision. If you are happy just listening to it, that's fine, but sometimes bigger is definitely better.

Today, many popular TV series love to show text messages as they occur on smartphones as part of an episode's storyline. It is obvious that the people behind this visual technique lack the understanding of low vision. By having a big enough screen, though, you will actually be able to make out what is written in the texted conversation appearing on the screen.

With the development of large flat-screen TVs, we now have many sizes from which to choose. The most common sizes are 32-, 43-, 55- and 65-inch screens. However, larger sizes such as 75-, 85- and even 98-inch models are also available. When buying any TV, keep in mind that the inch-screen size is measured from one corner of the screen diagonally up or down to the other corner.

Before buying a TV screen, go to the TV store that shows TVs turned on, so you can determine which size is right for your vision. Make sure you also know the allotted size of the space in your house where the TV will be located. Large screens can be hung on a wall or placed on stands to sit in or on a cabinet. There is no doubt that extra-large TVs cost more—however, the prices of big screen TVs have been reduced greatly over the years. Even so, it's easy enough to wait for them to go on sale.

TV SCREENS AS COMPUTER SCREENS

Most TV screens can also function as a computer screen. Your tech person can set this up for you. If you use your computer for business purposes, and you have low vision, then the cost for having the work done would be a tax deduction. Speak with your tax preparer about it for a fuller understanding of the process prior to your next tax return.

TV REMOTE CONTROLS

If you struggle to use the TV remote because of low vision, here are some ways to cope. Put a red dot on the most commonly used settings. Perhaps, the MUTE and ON/OFF buttons. You can also use a large button remote sold on the internet. It will need to be compatible with your TV brand. You can also set your smartphone or voice-activated assistant to turn your TV on, change channels, adjust the volume, and so on.

SPORTS

If you are a sports fan, you may have difficulty watching sports on TV. Not all sports are easy to watch. Some sports, like tennis and golf, are especially hard to watch because the balls are small and hard to follow when hit hard. You may be able to see football, basketball, and soccer better because the balls are larger and don't travel as fast.

If watching games still frustrates you, even though you have a large screen, you may consider turning off the sound of your TV and turning on a radio broadcast as you watch. Radio sports announcers provide a much greater description of all the plays since they are broadcasting to their listeners and not to a TV audience.

READING

The act of reading is important because it entertains you, provides you with helpful information, and stimulates your brain. Reading is a wonderful way to escape reality and stress and to improve your life. And while you may have enjoyed reading all your life, now you may find it a struggle or even impossible to read words in print. The good news is that you can still "read," but in different ways.

In this section, we will share lots of ways that you can still "read." Some ways are free, while others may carry a monthly charge.

LARGE-PRINT BOOKS

Many of the better-selling popular titles are published in large-print editions for low-vision readers. In fact, your library probably has a whole section of large-print books that you can access for free with a library card. You can also buy large-print books online. Be aware that they normally cost more than their original print editions.

There is also the option of using a magnification device to increase the size of the copy on each page. (See Chapter 13, *Magnification Options*, page 233.)

EBOOKS

Almost every book that is published today is also available in an ebook format. This is the electronic version of the printed edition that can be read on smartphones, tablets, and computers. The words flow on the screen to fit the size of the screen. For those with low vision, the reader can increase the letter size of the words until the copy is readable.

Ebooks can be purchased online for viewing on a smartphone, tablet, or computer. They can also be rented or purchased through many online services—or you can get ebooks through your library. Check with your local library to set up an account.

BOOKS ON TAPE

Today, while there are a number of other options to listen to books being read aloud, audiobooks are still available on cassette tapes. All you need is a recorder to play them. These audiobooks can be purchased online, in stores, or taken out from libraries.

For libraries that continue to provide a books-on-tape program for the visually impaired, the service works as follows: The library sends you an information sheet for you to list your interests and favorite authors. You will also need to have a form signed by your eye doctor or a librarian that your vision is low. After you return this form to the library, they will send you a free tape player and several tapes of 4 to 5 books each that will interest you.

The National Library Service for the Blind and Print Disabled (NLS) also provides free cassette players and tapes to hundreds of thousands of books, magazines, and music materials. (See *Resources*, page 308.)

While many libraries still maintain this service, advances in technology have made the process of listening to books much simpler. In many cases, digital audiobooks—set up as MP3 sound files rather than cassettes or compact discs and offered most popularly to date by Audible.com—have replaced books on tape.

AUDIBLE BOOKS, NEWSPAPERS, AND MAGAZINES

The ability to record books, newspapers, and magazines digitally and make them available as downloads from the internet has been a game changer, especially for people who have low vision or are blind. These audible editions can be listened to on your smartphone, tablet, and computer. When hooked up correctly, you can have Amazon's Alexa play the digital audiobook file from their Audible.com anywhere that you have a speaker in your home.

Audible books are available on many online services. For example, Amazon offers an Audible Library service. For one monthly subscription fee, you can order and then listen to any available audiobooks that interest you. In addition, many newspapers and magazines are available in a narrated format. They can be purchased directly from the publication, or from online services such as Google Play.

The National Library Service for the Blind and Print Disabled provides a similar service for the blind and those with low vision. This service is called BARD, Blind and Print Disabled Braille and Audio Reading

Download. It provides instant access to hundreds of thousands of books, magazines, and music materials in audio and electronic braille (ebraille) for free. (See *Resources*, page 308.)

If you miss reading your favorite magazines, you can also have some magazines and podcasts (see below) read aloud to you either by Alexa or on your smartphone.

NON-AUDIO MAGAZINES, E-NEWSLETTERS, AND NEWSPAPERS

Many of us have favorite periodicals that may still only appear in print or digital formats. For some, using a magnifying device of one sort or another enables us to read printed copy. Because most of these periodicals are now available on the internet as individual articles, technology provides us with two other options. You can magnify the image on the screen in order to read it, or you can have it read to you out loud.

By bringing up the article on your screen, you can have the screen reader setting read the article aloud. Of course, while it may not sound like it's coming from a professional reader, it will at least provide you with the text in a clear and understandable manner. It is likely that over time, Artificial Intelligence (AI) will make it sound like it is being read by a professional. For now, though, it works reasonably well.

Now you see that there are lots of different ways a person with low vision or blindness can still "read." So, choose the service that's best for you and then curl up and enjoy a good read.

MUSIC

If you enjoy music, listening to your favorite songs may brighten your day. On top of that, listening to music has been shown to reduce anxiety, blood pressure, and pain. It also improves your sleep, mood, mental alertness, and memory. Now, reaping all those benefits by doing something enjoyable is pretty amazing!

However, for some of us, finding the music we love may not be all that easy for any number of reasons. Fortunately, modern technology once again saves the day. By going to your favorite internet search engine, you can locate the websites, radio stations, and/or YouTube channels that play the types of music you want to hear—from rock 'n roll to jazz to classical, it's practically all there.

Once you have learned the locations of these music channels on any of your devices, you can then simply instruct your voice-activated smartphone, tablet, or computer to go to your favorite music channel. For example, if you ask Alexa to play "America, the

Beautiful," then that is what "she" will do. Or just about any type of music you wish to hear.

To have access to even more music you can pay a low monthly fee to play songs from Alexa's music library called Amazon Music Unlimited, which has a catalog of over 100 million songs. So, you can access almost any song or artist. Or, you can become a member of BARD, the NLS Braille and Audio Reading Download service, which can provide you access to music for free. (To learn more about these services, see *Resources,* page 302.)

If you love to dance, choose suitable music, stand in one place, and get moving! Enjoy the beat and music. Your brain will thank you because it thrives on rhythm!

PODCASTS

Podcasts have become a very popular form of audio entertainment. In some ways they are like a radio show and they are perfect for people with low vision. They are available to listen to any time of the day or night, and the selections are seemingly endless. For example, there are more than 2.5 million podcasts available from Apple alone.

There are many different types of podcasts available. There are interview podcasts where a host interviews someone who is an expert on the topic.

There are podcasts where only one person talks on a particular topic. Storytelling podcasts tell a funny, informative, or scary story, or a cast of actors perform a theatrical production, and so many more. You are bound to find one or more that you enjoy.

To find a podcast you may wish to listen to, go to your preferred search engine on your smartphone or computer and ask to find a podcast based on your favorite subject. There are also many general and specialized apps that provide podcasts as well. Once you find a few podcasts that you enjoy listening to, it's easy to get hooked.

PUZZLES

If you used to enjoy the challenge of bringing together hundreds of pieces in jigsaw puzzles, you will be pleased to know that there are also puzzles made specifically for people with low vision. They have large pieces, but fewer than you will find in a standard puzzle. There are also large-print versions of Sudoku, crossword puzzles, and a number of other word games available for your amusement.

Many of these games can be found free online. If you have difficulty seeing them on your screen, simply increase the size of the image. Try one and see if it is challenging enough for you.

CARDS AND GAMES

If you enjoy playing cards but can no longer see their numbers and suits, there are playing cards specifically designed for you that are easier to read. You can find these decks of cards in one of the low-vision catalogs. (See *Resources*, page 335.)

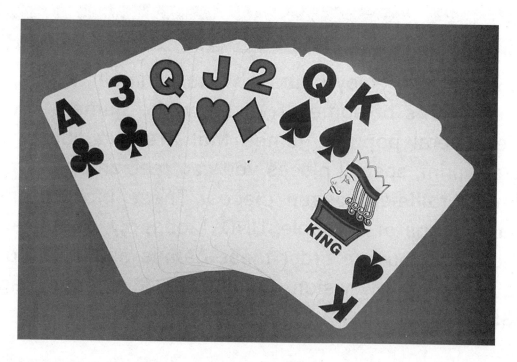

Playing cards that have large bold characters enable people with low vision to continue to participate in board games and card games.

You can use these cards to play solitaire or card games with friends. If you are blind, but you can read braille, there are special cards for you as well. These cards look like regular playing cards but have braille characters on each. When one of the sighted persons plays a card, they say aloud what card it is. For example, "Ace of spades." Of course, the person with no vision has to remember the cards that have been already played—but it can definitely sharpen your memory skills.

GAMES

You can also enjoy hours of entertainment with special editions of some of your favorite games. There are several popular games that are available with larger print, special pieces you can feel, and/or sometimes braille-embossed pieces. These include special editions of Scrabble, UNO, Monopoly, chess, and checkers. You can order these games online or from catalogs for low vision. Enjoy! (See *Resources*, page 335.)

PETS

Pets can bring you hours of joy, companionship, and love. They will often sit on your lap, cozy up at your feet, or even keep you company in bed. You can talk to them about anything, and they never disagree!

Of course, pets require a good deal of care. If you

live alone, you need to be sure you can take on the responsibilities that come along with having a pet—from daily feedings, exercise for the pet, grooming as needed, veterinarian visits, and the costs incurred for all of this care. Cats may be easier because all you will need to have is a litter box, while you need to take a dog outside to do his business. And you will also need to be sure you have enough pet food on hand. It is something to think about.

If you live with someone who is willing to share the necessary tasks with you, then owning and loving a pet together can be a neat experience.

Vision-impaired owners of dogs may struggle with cleaning up after a dog who has done his business outside. But keep in mind that totally blind persons who have guide dogs have this method of pet care, which should work for you. When you take your dog out, notice when he stops and squats down. Without distracting the animal too much, gently place your hand on the dog's back. If it is straight, then the dog is just peeing. However, if the dog is taking a poop, his back is normally in a crouched curve. Then you just have your hand follow the dog's back further down to the ground, where you should be ready to scoop up the poop with a plastic bag when the dog has finished.

If you let your dog go out in a fenced backyard to

do his business, there are actually pooper-scooper services available in many cities that come to your home to remove the waste from your yard.

One more thing to consider. As mentioned in Chapter 3, pets can also be a tripping hazard. If your floors are dark and your pet has dark fur, he may blend into the floor. You may not see the pet, and you can trip over him. Or, if your animal has blond or white fur, you might not see them on a light-colored floor. Perhaps a contrasting-colored or fluorescent collar might help. There are even collars that light up at night. You may als consider using a collar that produces a sound, in addition to being bright.

CONCLUSION

In this chapter, we have discussed the many ways you can enjoy yourself at home. You should make it a point to find activities that make you happy and joyful each day. In the next chapter, we will discuss ways to leave your home and enjoy your community, go to stores, and keep appointments.

7

Traveling Outside Your Home

For some people, low vision tends to limit their desire to get out of their home. In their home, they know how to get around and where the things they need are located. And why not? At home, they feel comfortable and safe in their familiar surroundings. But in a real sense, they are also cutting themselves off from the rest of the world.

While initially getting out of the house may cause some anxiety, it also provides an important part of our personal freedom. Freedom to connect with people, nature, and your community. To get together with relatives and friends, or to meet with your doctor, dentist, barber, or hairdresser. As you will discover, getting out of your home or apartment will raise your spirits. The more you venture out of your home, the more likely you will want to try different activities.

In this chapter, we will start with something simple—just walking about in your neighborhood. Next, we will discuss how to find transportation for free or minimal charges. Third, we will consider getting out to shop. Finally, we will suggest going to community events that might interest you.

WALKING

Sitting outside in a chair in your yard, if you have one, can be relaxing and enjoyable. Or you may just want to take a walk to chat with neighbors or enjoy Mother Nature. All these activities will lift your mood, relieve stress, and improve your sleep. It's also a great exercise that can improve your mental and physical health. If you live near a park, walk to the park and enjoy the peacefulness of the scenery, even if you can't see it clearly. Listen to the birds and smell the fresh air.

If you have enough remaining vision to see any steps up or down outside your home, the location of the sidewalks, and any obstacles that may be in your pathway, then you may want to take short walks. Remember that safety is always a first priority. The rule of thumb is if you do not feel safe walking a route or crossing a street by yourself, then do not try it.

But sometimes low vision comes with the fear of tripping over a crack in the sideway or getting lost. These are certainly real concerns, but there are things you can do to help diminish these fears and allow you to move around safely and independently. These aids include orientation and mobility training, walking companions (sighted guides), sunglasses, long canes, and a dog guide.

ORIENTATION AND MOBILITY (O&M) TRAINING

The two things someone with low vision or blindness must be aware of when traveling outdoors is their location (known as *orientation*) and their knowledge of travel (called *mobility*)—that is, how to get to their destination. If you have never had any orientation and mobility training, then you may lack the confidence to take a walk in your own neighborhood. O&M training can help with mobility skills and confidence. That is a very common feeling. For those who have received or will receive O&M training, you should soon notice that you walk with much more confidence and safety after the training. (See Chapter 11, *Helpful Aids for Those Who Are Blind*, page 193.)

WALKING COMPANIONS

If you still cannot walk safely because of your vision, ask a person to be your walking companion to act as a sighted guide. They could be a relative, a friend, or a neighbor. They may need some help in order to be a good sighted guide. (See Chapter 11, *Helpful Aids for Those Who Are Blind*, page 193.)

There may also be local volunteer groups that provide sighted guides.

CHOOSING SUNGLASSES

Many eye doctors recommend their patients wear sunglasses/filters outside to protect their eyes from further damage. Some colors of sunglasses can be more helpful than others. It is an individual's choice. Since no two people are the same, make sure to try out different types of sunglasses. It is the best way to determine what works best. Here are some suggestions on how to purchase one that is best for you:

■ Fit-over filters will fit over your existing eyeglasses. These types of sunglasses are nice since they are much larger and allow you to use your regular prescription eyeglasses. If you do not wear eyeglasses, then find a pair of regular sunglasses that you feel comfortable putting on.

■ There are many shades of filters such as amber, yellow, green, and gray. Each of these colors have variants that are darker or lighter. What this means is that there are many to choose from. The best way to test them all out is with an optometrist if that is possible for you.

ACCESSIBLE PEDESTRIAN SIGNALS (APS)

Some communities are starting to install devices with buttons attached to light poles at intersections that, when pressed, will tell you aloud when to walk safely, and how much time you have to cross. The official name for these devices is Accessible Pedestrian Signals or APS. Take a friend and try out newly installed devices in your neighborhood, so you understand how they work, so you might be able to use them alone.

TRANSPORTATION

Sometimes the easiest way for a person with low vision to get from point A to point B is to get a ride. Rides come in many forms. If you live in an urban area, rides are usually easier to come by. If you live in a rural area, you may have fewer options. By knowing what all your options are ahead of time, you can make sure you will get where you need to go on time. Here are several considerations. Some are free and others are not.

PUBLIC TRANSPORTATION

In urban areas, buses and trains are common modes of getting around. However, for people with low vision, these modes of transportation have a number of obstacles—from having to overcome steps to having to hold on to poles or overhead rails as a train or bus moves forward. While this may be a challenge for one person with low vision, it is less of a challenge if that person is accompanied by a sighted guide. Also, many cities offer reduced rates for those with a physical disability.

Your local public transportation system may also offer a door-to-door system for a small fee. This will require you to sign up for this program with documentation from a professional stating you need the door-to-door service.

As mentioned, public transportation can be difficult, but with the right help, it can be an option.

CAR RIDES FROM RELATIVES, FRIENDS, AND OTHERS

Perhaps you can pool together a network of relatives, friends, and neighbors who have cars and who have some free time to take you out to eat, shop, and go to appointments. Perhaps a neighbor goes shopping once a week. Ask if you can come along to do your own shopping. They might enjoy the company.

If you have a number of people to ask, you don't have to rely on just one person. Set up a schedule accordingly among the group. On the other hand, if you are lucky enough to have one person drive around, you could offer to pay for gas. You might also consider hiring a college student to come by to pick you up at fixed times.

COMMUNITY TRANSPORTATION OPTIONS

Community groups in your area may also offer transportation. For example, many communities have a small bus to take senior or disabled people to appointments for a small charge or free. If needed, the driver will assist you on and off the bus. Your place of worship may also have a van to take you to services.

CAR RIDE SERVICES

Taxicabs can also transport you for a fee. One advantage is if you deal with a small cab company you may be able to ask for a specific driver on a given date. One disadvantage of taxis is that riders and drivers may smoke in the vehicle, which you may find offensive. If not, it shouldn't be a problem.

Another option is using Uber or Lyft. These businesses operate vehicles that should be smoke-free. Another advantage is they may be a little cheaper than a cab. Their drivers are most often courteous, friendly, and helpful and will be glad to assist you if you have disabilities.

You can order an Uber or a Lyft on your iPhone or Android by installing an Uber or Lyft app. Ask someone you trust to enter your credit card number, your home address, and addresses of places you commonly go. You can choose to pay with cash by going to their app ahead of time.

CAN YOU STILL DRIVE YOUR CAR?

Initially, it would seem that low vision would disqualify people from legally being able to drive a car. However, most states have some flexibility for those with vision impairments. For an individual with low vision to obtain a driver's license, here are some general requirements:

■ Drivers may need approximately 20/70 vision and a wide field of sight to qualify.

■ Drivers may be restricted to driving only during the day, and not during the night.

■ A conditional driver's license that may require driver training, scheduled updates, and reports from an optometrist or ophthalmologist.

■ Passable vision in one eye and visual impairment in the other eye.

Then to order a driver just tap the address where you want to go and your phone will let you know how soon your driver will arrive, the model and color of the car, and its license plate number. Ubers often have small signs on the windshield identifying them as

---

■ Use of vision aids, such as bioptic or telescopic lenses. (See Chapter 13, *Magnification Options*, page 233 and *Resources*, page 311 to learn more about bioptic telescopic glasses.)

Drivers will normally have to participate in a special drivers' training program to learn how to use the telescopic or bioptic lenses while driving. Bioptics are prescribed by a licensed optometrist or ophthalmologist.

The bottom line is that, even with low vision, given the rules in your state, you may still be able to drive a car. However, there are still a number of things to consider. Do you live in a heavily trafficked area or in a rural location? Is driving your only means to get to a specific location? Do you still feel safe behind the wheel of your car? It is not easy giving up your driver's license, but it is a decision you may have to make. Just make sure it's the right one.

Uber or Lyft. However, it is likely that you may not be able to read the sign or the license plate.

Because of this—and for your safety—when your driver arrives, check to be sure it's your Uber or Lyft by asking the driver what your name is. They should have that info readily at hand and are supposed to call you by name when you get in and know where your destination is. If he or she doesn't know your name or your destination, don't get in!

After you have arrived at your destination, your fare is automatically charged to your card, or you may pay in cash if you indicate that on your app. You can choose to tip or not to tip, and you can rate your driver. However, you must check ahead of time to see if the riding service you use accepts cash payments. In some cities and towns, cash payments are not accepted. This is done for the safety of the drivers.

SHOPPING

In-person shopping can be very frustrating for people with low vision. In groceries, pharmacies, and other retail stores, the aisles are often marked high above the ends of the aisle (endcaps) with signs indicating the items in that aisle. These may be difficult to see. In addition, the individual prices of products and expiration dates may be even harder to read. A simple solution would be to shop with someone who can direct you to the right area of the store and the aisle where your product is located. He or she can also help you read labels and prices on items.

If you shop alone, you can use your assistive device such as a handheld magnifier to identify and read aloud labels of items you may want to buy. Some stores can offer an employee to shop with you and provide one-on-one shopping assistance. Call ahead to find out if they offer such a service. Of course, once you are familiar with the store, you may be able to find what you need yourself.

RELIGIOUS SERVICES

If you would like to attend religious services at a church, synagogue, or mosque, you may now hesitate to do so because it may be hard to get there. Be aware that many places of worship offer transportation to pick up physically disabled worshipers. Call ahead to see if they do. You may also be apprehensive about walking into a room full of people you can no longer recognize. Here again, you might consider calling ahead and talking with someone in charge who can make an effort to see if there is someone there to meet you and help get you seated. Or, you might ask a friend who attends another house of worship to take you along and introduce you to his or her friends.

These places of worship often have large-print hymnals, bibles, programs, or other religious materials available for you. Ask the usher if there are any such books available. Taking along your lighted LED magnifying glass will also help. If you are having difficulty seeing what is going on, just relax and enjoy the music, the message, and the camaraderie of the people sharing the services. Through this place of worship there may be activities you would enjoy—meals to share or other events that reach out to help your community.

COMMUNITY EVENTS

Communities, depending upon their size, often offer events you may wish to attend provided they match your interests. If local politics interest you, attend city council, parks and recreation meetings, school board events, or even a criminal or civil trial open to the public. Find what interests you.

There may be all kinds of community-sponsored musical events you could share with a friend. Your city may have a symphony orchestra with several scheduled concerts. Or there may be outdoor band concerts in the warm months. There may be outdoor facilities for open-air productions. Plays and concerts put on by local groups or interesting seminars at colleges could also be available. The opportunities may be endless in your town, it's just a matter of identifying a few you would enjoy. You will find that many of these events are free or are reasonably priced. Call or go online to your local chamber of commerce for more information and ideas.

CONCLUSION

Perhaps it's just a walk around the block, or maybe it's a trip to a doctor. Do not be afraid to take someone with you. You don't have to do it alone. And the more you do it, the better you will feel both emotionally and physically.

You should not allow the fear of going outside to take hold. If you take the time to understand how important it is, you can overcome this fear. Yes, you need to properly prepare to take those trips outside, but it will be worth it.

8

Reading and Writing with Low Vision

For most of us, the ability to read and write has allowed us to carry on our daily routines. However, when we start to lose our eyesight, the act of reading and writing becomes more challenging. We often turn to electronic devices to help us communicate with others. Based on the level of our low vision, the use of these devices allows us to control how we can read words or write to others.

In previous chapters, we have discussed some of the new devices that are available to help people with low vision to read and communicate with others. In this chapter, we will provide you with a closer look at the controllable options already in your computer that may help you write and read. The following are some basic options and settings that can make this process of reading and writing easier for you when you are typing or reading on your computer, tablet, or smartphone devices. It's up to you to choose the formats that work best for you.

READING AND WRITING

We are all taught to read and write at a relatively early age. By the time we finish school, we take these skills for granted. However, when we start to lose our eyesight, the act of reading and writing becomes more difficult. We often turn to electronic forms when communicating with others. Based on the level of our low vision, the use of these electronic devices allows us to control how we can read words or write to others. The following are some basic options you have to make this process of reading and writing easier for you.

FONTS

The style of a printed letter and its matching numbers, punctuations, and symbols is called a *font*. There are literally hundreds of fonts that are available on any computer and smartphone device. When you are choosing fonts for reading or writing, how do you know what to choose?

The answer is relatively simple. You want a font made up of letters that are easy to recognize and that stands out on the background they will appear on. There are a number of factors to consider when choosing the right font for you. These include type style, kerning, size, leading, boldface, and capital letters.

Type Styles

There are essentially two styles of fonts. One is called *serif* and the other is *non-serif,* also known as *sans-serif.*

■ **Serif.** The word serif refers to a font with little extra squiggles added to each character. For example, a commonly used font is Times New Roman which looks like this:

This is an example of Times New Roman.

The extra tiny squiggles or "feet" or "tails" on each letter makes it a serif font. These squiggles make this font harder to read if you have low vision.

■ **Non-Serif/Sans-Serif.** This style of font contains no squiggles. They are composed solely of plain straight and curved lines. Here are three different types of non-Serif font styles—Tahoma, Arial, and Helvetica:

This is an example of Tahoma.

This is an example of Arial.

This is an example of Helvetica.

Each of these non-Serif fonts look very similar—clean and simple, but there is another factor to consider as well.

Kerning

If you look carefully at these three fonts, you will notice that they differ in the space between each letter. This space is referred to as *kerning*. Some fonts provide more space than others. The more space between letters can make a big difference when reading and writing.

For smartphones, you cannot adjust the kerning of letters on the available font styles, unless you create your own set of fonts. It is easier to find a font with decent kerning between the letters. On computer programs there is usually a setting that can adjust the kerning to make it easier for you to use.

Font Sizes

The *point size* of the font you use is just as important. The size on most devices is adjustable and is located in the display settings on your smartphone or the box next to the font description on your word processor. Here are some examples of sizes you could choose:

12 pt This is the most commonly used size for normal vision.

14 pt This is an example of 14 pt.

16 pt This is an example of 16 pt.

18 pt. This is an example of 18 pt.

20 pt. This is an example of 20 pt.

Leading

The space between lines can also play a role in your ability to read copy clearly. The technical name given to this space is called *leading*. Line spacing can be adjusted to allow each line to have enough space above it and below it for easier reading. Most devices have standard line space settings that will provide you with the following space between lines.

Single-spaced
1.5-spaced
Double-spaced

Along with the standard spacing, there is also a setting that allows you to customize the leading should you need to adjust the space more.

Boldface

Standard fonts come in normal and boldface type. Boldface type provides thicker lines for each letter.

This is not bolded. **This is bolded.**

It's important to know that each font style may have a different boldface thickness, which can make a difference. Normally, boldface is used to make a word or phrase stand out. For those with low vision, using boldface makes words easier to read.

All Capital Letters

If your low vision progresses, you may find it easier to use all capital letters as you write or type on your computer. When working on a Microsoft Word program on a computer, once you have capitalized all your words and completed your message, you can highlight the whole message, and turn your copy into an upper and lower case sentence structure, if you wish to send it off as an email or print the document. In the same way, you can copy the emails you receive and put them into your Word program, where you can enlarge the email and/or capitalize all the copy.

There are several settings on your computer that you can explore that may make it easier to see what you are typing or what you want to read. You should try setting up a whole page of copy and putting it into different-sized fonts, and leadings. Don't be afraid to experiment. Using any or all of these options, find a font and font size that makes reading easiest with you.

ADDITIONAL AIDS

There are a few other things you can do to see what else may improve your ability to read and write.

Color

The colors of the letters and the color of the background—whether they are on a screen or on paper—may also make the word easier to read or write with. Usually, black print on white paper or on computer screens is the most readable. However, the type of eye problem you may be experiencing can play a role in how well you see the words. Also, keyboards may be easier to use if the individual key's background is white and the letters and numbers are black. You might check in a computer store to see if a keyboard with black keys on white or white keys on black or even different-colored backgrounds improves your vision.

Overlays

When reading, printed material colored overlays (plastic sheets) can sometimes be used to help people see print more clearly. They are especially used for children with reading problems, but it may benefit a few adults as well. The overlays come in a variety of colors that you can buy online. Just place each color sheet over the page you want to read. Try doing this with a number of color sheets to see if there is any improvement. While it may not work for everyone, it is worth trying.

Magnification

For low-vision users, any magnification device—ranging from small portable handheld magnifiers to full-sized desktop low-vision machines to head-worn devices—may be used depending upon preference. Many users have more than one device or product to magnify what they want to read. (See Chapter 13, *Magnification Options*, page 233.)

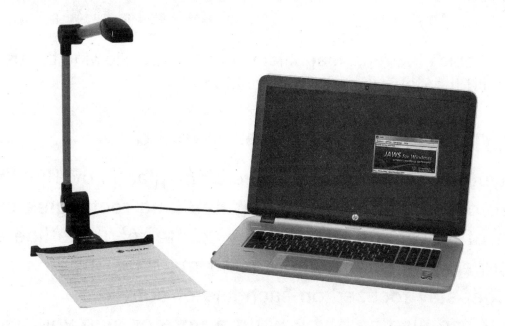

When connected to a Windows computer, the Pearl camera is used to capture an image of text and is then read aloud for the user.

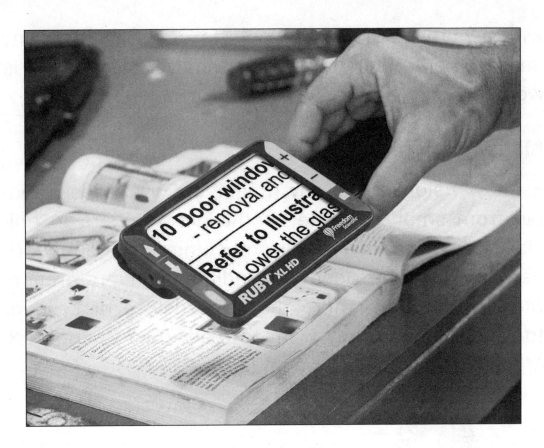

A portable electronic magnifier with a handle allowing the user to hold the device in various positions.

A Typoscope for Reading and Writing

A *typoscope* is an inexpensive black plastic overlay the size of a sheet of paper that has long rectangles cut out of it. These cutouts allow you to read one line at a time when placed on reading material. It helps the reader stay focused on each line of copy.

It can also help you write a note or sign your signature in a straight line. Whether you need to sign a check, write messages on greeting cards or envelopes, or pass on a note, using a typoscope can make it easier to write. They are available from a number of the catalog companies. (See *Resources*, page 335.)

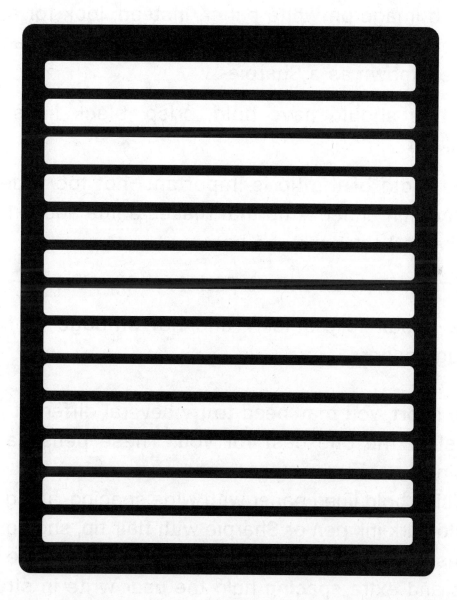

This type of writing aid is placed on top of a blank piece of paper. Each line of this aid is an open space, allowing the user to easily write within the spaces provided.

Using Pens or Pencils

When writing, pencils are probably not a good writing tool for you. In general, pencils do not produce a dark enough image on white paper. Instead, look for a flair tip pen that produces thicker lines—in particular, the gel pen known as a Sharpie.

■ Letters should have bold, crisp, black lines that stand out.

■ The width of the tip is important—not too wide but not too thin either. A tip that makes a line about 1 mm (millimeter) thick may be best.

■ Some low-vision writers prefer felt-tip pens.

■ Ink should dry quickly and not smudge or bleed through paper.

In short, you may need to try several different pens to select the one best for you. These pens can be obtained at office supply stores.

Using bold lined paper with wide spacing, along with a bold dark-ink pen or Sharpie with flair tip, should help the user write notes, grocery lists, and letters. The bold lines and extra spacing help the user write in straight lines. The bold lined paper may also be positioned under a low-vision machine camera while writing if magnification is needed.

Easily see and stay within the lines of this white double-sided bold lined paper. This paper is great for to-do lists, daily reminders, letters, and anything else you need.

WRITING USING YOUR VOICE

If the writing techniques we have discussed still represent a problem, you can also write using just your voice. Voice input or voice recognition is software that is now available almost everywhere. In the same way you can control your lights and television to go "ON" and "OFF" by stating a command out loud, you can create typed words on your computer, tablet, and smartphone.

To produce a document on your computer you can use your keyboard and mouse, your voice, or a combination of both. You will quickly discover that creating words with your voice is faster and even more accurate with modern technology improvements. Now, many devices come standard with voice-recognition software already included in the device. If it is not included, a third-party product can be obtained and installed to provide voice recognition.

After typing with a keyboard or with your voice, the text that is produced can be read aloud back to you, so you can make sure the text is accurate and reflects what you wanted to say. (See Chapter 14, *Software Reading Programs*, page 254.)

READING

Most people who are legally blind may have some remaining vision as has been mentioned in this book. Most persons who lose some vision later in life have read with their eyes for many years rather than with speech output. Many low-vision persons who are trying to read information on a screen (ranging from a small smartphone screen to a large computer screen) will need at least one or a combination of these built-in settings or additional software programs:

- Larger text

- Bolder text

- Easy-to-read font

- Preferred spacing

- Preferred foreground and background colors

- Optimal lighting in the room

When trying to read incoming information appearing in a digital format on a screen, in most cases, you should be able to change settings that allow for you to alter the text and change the spacing. All of the settings listed above can be customized for you on your computer or device.

The lighting on the device's screen can also be brightened with contrast changes using the Settings menu. Lamps in a room can be moved or changed to produce less glare on the screen for easier reading. Overhead lighting, coming from the ceiling, is often not optimal because of glare produced from the screen you are using. Experimenting with these settings is likely to be the most practical way for you to determine what works best for you.

For low-vision people trying to read information on paper—such as newspapers, magazines, and newsletters—they will need low-vision aids such as magnifying devices. (See Chapter 13, *Magnification Options*, page 233.) Some of these low-vision aids can make the text bigger, and add different color foreground and background. Again, lighting in the room is almost always a factor to consider.

Persons who are totally blind will need to depend upon speech to read information. If the information is printed on paper, the reader can scan the text with an OCR (Optical Character Recognition) device and the text will be read aloud. This also applies to the person with low vision.

If the information you want to read is already on the computer screen, you will need a software screen-reading program—either a program that comes with the computer or a third-party program you purchase. (See Chapter 14, *Software Reading Programs*, page 254.)

For persons who are good braille readers, you may connect a refreshable braille device to your computer or smartphone. Braille access for computers may work best for those users who are experienced braille users and can read it quickly. The information will be displayed on the braille device, and the words can also be spoken if that is preferable to the user.

CONCLUSION

Some of the information in this chapter may seem a bit technical, however, don't let that stop you from experimenting. Once you begin making these changes in your devices, you will quickly see that they will improve the way you read and write. These technological advances have truly changed the world for those with low vision, and blindness. Simply put, it reconnects you to your friends, relatives, and the rest of the world.

9

Your Money

You already know that managing and spending your money carefully is important—you want to conserve what you have and most likely increase the amount. To deal with the subject of money properly, we will be covering three areas. We will first discuss your personal finances. This includes managing expenses, investing wisely, and avoiding financial scams. To some, this may seem a bit overwhelming, but it is important to always keep track of your money.

Second, we will examine the job opportunities and careers that you may have had no idea existed for you despite your vision loss. We will consider just what jobs are available, what training and education you can receive free, and how to apply for a job you may want. As you will discover, advancements in technology have provided a gateway to many jobs that can provide a steady income, security, and even new friendships.

And third, if your income is limited and you feel you have few resources to turn to, we will look at the many programs designed to offer you the assistance

you may need. This includes financial help, health benefits, training to cope with your vision loss, and other
free resources provided by federal, state, and local
governments as well as from private organizations.
These agencies are in place to make your life easier by
helping you cope with your vision issues and helping
to ensure that you have sufficient financial income.
They want you to enjoy the best life you can.

PERSONAL FINANCES

Keeping your personal finances in good order is crucial for everyone. It can be time-consuming, confusing, frustrating, and anxiety-provoking even for sighted
persons. Those with impaired vision may struggle even
more. In this Personal Finances section, we will give
you tips for identifying the different bill denominations
of money in your wallet, special services available to
you from your bank, how to obtain special credit cards,
and more. We hope these tips will make handling your
finances easier and safer so you will have peace of
mind about this important aspect of your life.

IDENTIFYING THE BILLS IN YOUR POCKET

Is there anything more frustrating, yet extremely
important, than struggling to identify what money you

have in your pocket, wallet, or purse? Or what currency is handed back to you by a salesperson, bank teller, or anyone else in the midst of any "in person" financial transactions? We have several suggestions to help you with what seems like an easy task—but one that is so difficult for those with low vision.

Larger Numbers on the Bills

Most people are not aware that there is a large currency number printed on paper bills. That number can be found on the back lower right-hand corner of $5, $10, $20, $50, and $100 bills. This is specifically done to help people with low vision identify the bill. It is definitely worth checking out.

The Right Fold

For those who cannot see the numbers on these bills, there is the classic system of folded money. Ask a trusted person to help you with this folding method for keeping paper money straight in your wallet or purse. First, keep your $1 bills unfolded. Second, fold $5 bills in half lengthwise. Third, fold $10 bills in half by width. Fourth, fold $20 bills in half both lengthwise and then by width—as shown in the accompanying photograph. This makes them easier to feel for in your wallet or placed in a pocket.

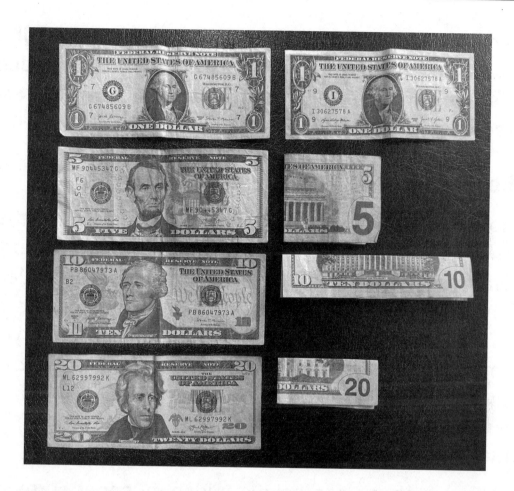

To organize and recognize currency in a wallet, a low-tech folding method may be used. It is tactile and easy to use: $1 bill can be flat; $5 bill in half crosswise; $10 bill in half lengthwise; and $20 bill like the $10 bill and then half again like the $5 bill. Or you can use your own method.

Click Pocket or Money Brailler

If you use braille, a gadget called the Click Pocket or Money Brailler helps identify a denomination by putting the edge of the bill into this small device, which then prints the denomination in braille that can be felt and read. After identifying the denomination of the bill, it can be folded down and put away until it is needed. This item is available from the catalog MaxiAids (See *Resources*, page 336.)

The Currency Reader

Another small device is a bill currency reader that announces the value of any U.S. currency through *vibrations*. If you are a U.S. citizen or national resident with low vision or blindness, then this is available to you free from the U.S. Bureau of Engraving once you complete and submit an application. (See *Resources*, page 324.)

Smartphone Identification

Your smartphone can help you identify paper currency using various apps. Most of these apps are free and can identify both U.S. and foreign currencies. They use text-to-speech and are able to read a bill and tell you out loud the denomination. In most cases, Wi-Fi is not required for them to work:

■ Apple offers a Cash Reader Money app, which scans and identifies paper bills.

■ Google Play provides the Cash Reader app to scan and identify paper bills.

■ If you have an Android smartphone, there are two apps available for use. One is called the Ideal Currency Identifier, which identifies only U.S. currency, and the other is the MCT app, which also identifies foreign money.

■ Microsoft's Seeing AI app on Android phones or an iPhone can identify not only currency, but it can also recognize people, read text, scan barcodes, and even describe any form of physical scenery that may be directly in front of you!

IDENTIFYING COINS

Have you noticed that the U.S. Mint makes coins with two identifying features you can feel? One feature is the size and thickness of a coin. The second feature is the texture of its outer ridge, which you can feel with your fingernail. Pennies and nickels have smooth edges, with nickels being the larger of the two. A dime is smaller and thinner than other coins and has rough or ridged edges. Quarters and half-dollars also have ridges with quarters being larger in size than dimes, nickels, and pennies. Half-dollars are larger than the previous coins and have ridged edges. Finally, silver dollar coins are the largest coins and have rough edges. Try practicing with a handful of coins until you can easily identify them.

KEEPING TRACK OF YOUR FINANCES

If you have someone you trust to keep tabs on your finances—from paying bills to keeping track of your income—you definitely have a lot less to worry about. For many people with low vision, however, that responsibility falls squarely on their own shoulders. While the process can be somewhat stressful, you should be fine if you set up a routine that helps you take care of your financial responsibilities.

In the next section, we will first discuss the elements involved in taking care of your recurring expenses, and then we'll offer some thoughts on finding the right places to invest your savings. It is important to keep in mind that there are people out there who are looking to take advantage of you—perhaps even more so, if you have low vision. If something sounds too good to be true, then it's probably not.

ORGANIZING YOUR DESK

Let's begin at the place where you take care of your daily expenses—your desk. For persons who do not often use digitized information on a computer, organizing your desk or a table where you will do your financial paperwork may be a helpful first step. Try to have everything together you use frequently—stamps, envelopes, scissors, return address labels, your personal checks, and deposit slips.

You want the especially bright and strong illumination that comes from what is called *task lighting*—a setup that shines light directly down on the paperwork you want to view. You may need a handheld magnifier or other devices that magnify what you are viewing. If magnification does not provide enough assistance, you may need a device that will scan the paper and read it aloud for you. (See Chapter 14, *Software Reading Programs*, page 254 and *Resources*, page 329.)

Having differently colored folders to hold different types of paperwork may help you keep things in order. For example, a red folder could hold medical reports and test results, a black folder could hold bills that need continually prompt payment, a green folder for papers needed to pay your taxes, and so on. In addition, you might consider using fluorescent colored Post-it notes to tag important pages and files. Storing these paper files in areas that are easy to access is important as well.

If you struggle to add up columns of numbers, just buy a pad of large-print graph paper that has large squares. Then put a digit of each number in its own square. Then add up the columns. You can also ask your smartphone, computer, or Alexa to add up the numbers for you.

PAYING BILLS

Paying bills is not a fun task for anyone. But for someone with low vision, it can be especially difficult and frustrating. It is, however, important that it is taken care of at all times. There are essentially two ways to take care of paying your bills. There is the traditional way of receiving paper bills and sending off checks, and then there is the "paperless" approach that most large companies now encourage.

Paying the Traditional Way

First, you sort out the bills from the rest of your mail. You then open the envelope, remove the invoice, and look for the amount owed and the date that it is due. This may require a magnification device to read what the bill is for as you go through these documents. Once done, you write the check or get a money order and mail it out. As you make your payments, you also need to keep track of the bills you've paid. That can be done on your computer, or a form you keep on or near your desk.

That system works fine for many people, but modern technology has greatly changed the way people now pay their bills. There are now better and easier ways to accomplish this task.

Paying Bills Online

By using a secure internet line, most bills can be paid online. What this means is that instead of getting a paper bill mailed to you, you will get the bill sent to you as an email. Of course, you will need a screen that can enlarge the information or talking software to read it to you. Given this approach, you normally have three ways to pay these online bills—either by credit card, debit card, or taken out directly from your bank account.

With recurring monthly bills, you can set up any of these three ways to pay. The good news is that most, if not all, of these monthly payments may be set up on an automatic basis. Once this type of payment sched-ule has been set up, you will receive a bill emailed to you each month followed by another email telling you that the bill has been paid.

The problem with using a credit card is that, if it is compromised, the credit card company will need to issue you a new card. Then you have to update the new card info for every online account you have, which is a pain! Instead, use your bank account's checking and routing numbers. You can find them both at the bottom of each check. You or a helper can enter these numbers into the online accounts for your utilities, businesses, and so on. You or your helper will need to watch your email account for new bills so you can pay them on time.

WORKING WITH YOUR BANK

Banks today have a number of ways to assist their vision-impaired clients. This is due to the fact that banks have a legal obligation to make reasonable policies and practices for people with low vision so they can use their banking services. To find out what policies and products your bank offers, introduce yourself in person to the bank manager and/or staff. Try to call ahead to set up a meeting.

Choose a time when the bank is not busy. Try to avoid Friday afternoons, Saturdays, last days of the month, and lunch hours. Then keep in touch with one of the bankers by phone or in person to establish a relationship. You may need a trusted relative or friend to go with you. In some cases, you can have your relative or friend stay with you at the meeting, and in other cases, you might ask them to wait outside the manager's office until you are through. It all depends on the extent of your need for privacy.

Banks should have various services for their customers. For example, both Bank of America and Chase Bank—two of the larger American banks—offer free consumer and small business checking, savings, credit card, brokerage, and mortgage account statements, along with various other documents made available in large-print formats, audio, and braille. Your own bank may have similar services, so call or go online to see what services they offer their low-vision customers. If you find their services inadequate for your needs, find a bank that will work with your particular financial and visual needs.

OPENING BANK ACCOUNTS

Federal law requires that low-vision customers must be able to open a bank account and have guaranteed access to all available services. You can open an account in your name alone, or with some trusted relative or friend. If you request, the bank branch manager must read to you the rules of business and other terms and conditions in the presence of a witness. The bank manager must also inform you of your rights and liabilities before opening the account. You may ask that your account be clearly marked in all bank records with the words, "The account holder is visually impaired."

At this meeting, you can also discuss your banking needs such as large-print checks and monthly statements in braille, large print, audio, and/or online formats. You may want to have a trusted sighted relative's name listed along with your own on the checks, so they can write out checks if you are disabled. They can also receive duplicate statements so they can check on your behalf for fraudulent checks.

You can also apply for a special credit card designed for low-vision customers. You could set up a check deposit feature using an app on your smartphone. Then you just take a picture of your check and send it to your bank to be deposited. To set this up, you will need your home Wi-Fi code and Social Security number for your bank. Finally, ask who to contact if you have banking problems or questions. Keep that information in a convenient place.

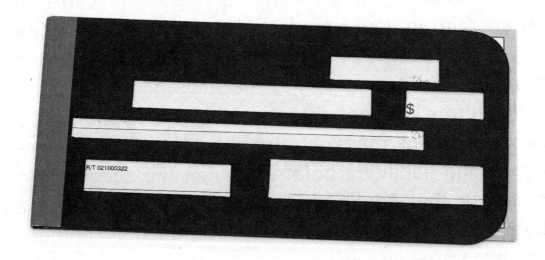

Guides like the one pictured here have slots so that the user can fill in the information where it should be written.

If you struggle to write a check because you can't see the different lines or boxes, there are check templates available in a number of catalogs. (See *Resources*, page 355). These devices fit over your check and have spaces where you can feel where you write the name of the person you are paying, the amount in dollars, a space to write the amount in words, a memo line, and a place for your signature (see photo on the facing page). Your bank may have one available that fits the design of your bank's checks.

CHECK DEPOSITS

To deposit a check, you have several options. First, you could use a lighted magnifier to see the check or scanning device to read it aloud. After confirming what the check states, you can endorse it, and if you want, you may write the amount in a large-print account (register) book that you can buy online or get free from your bank. You can then use this book/register to record the checks you write and the checks you deposit.

At the end of the month, you can compare your balance with your bank's balance. You want to be sure no one is writing checks on your account you haven't approved. After endorsing a check, take it to your bank with your deposit slip. If you own a smartphone with an app from your bank, you can easily deposit your check by taking a picture of the check and following the directions on your bank app. With this method in place, there is no need to travel to a bank branch.

Another option is to have any paychecks, dividend checks, and other forms of payment that you are due deposited automatically to your bank account. You can then check your account online to make sure the right amount was deposited.

CREDIT CARDS

How does a low-vision or blind person use a credit card? First, if you are going to have more than one, choose different colors and patterns for each card. Also, credit, debit, and ATM cards are available with braille labels.

The dots allow you to feel the difference if you are severely vision-impaired.

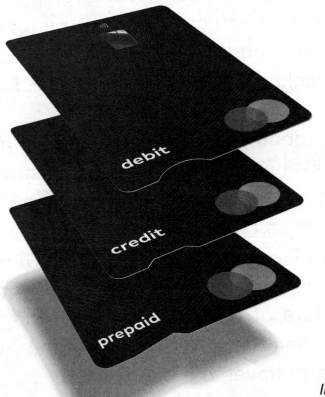

Touch Card™ credit cards have a round notch, the debit card has a squarish notch, and the prepaid card has a triangular notch.

Image courtesy of Mastercard International Incorporated.

Some credit card companies make cards with different shapes for low-vision people who can feel the differences. For example, the card on the facing page is from Mastercard—it is called the Touch Card™ and features differently shaped notches on one edge—rounded for debit, squared for credit, and triangular for prepaid. Other cards have embossed numbers or raised letters that can be felt with your fingers.

Your monthly credit card statement probably comes to you printed in small words and numbers that most regular customers struggle to see. You could read these aloud using OrCam, in large print online, or on your smartphone. The bank or credit card company that issues the card should also be able to provide you with large-print statements.

PAYING TAXES

For those who are sight-impaired, preparing to pay federal and state income taxes, property taxes, and other local taxes can take a lot of work. It requires that you have all the right paperwork in-hand and that you know how to fill out all the necessary tax forms correctly. There are normally two ways to get this job done. You can do it yourself, or you can work with an accountant. Both require you to have all the necessary paperwork and forms available.

ORGANIZING YOUR PAPERWORK

If you are one of those folks who already has a system in place for putting away your tax information through-out any given year, congratulations! If not, then having the right folder system in place will help. For example,

---

SCAMMERS & FRAUDSTERS & THIEVES, OH MY!

Over the last few years, the internet has become home to people with one intention—to steal your money, and your assets. In many cases, this is done by computer hackers who are able to steal your personal information such as your Social Security and credit card numbers, your driver's license infor-mation, your banking information, and your home address. Unfortunately, this can be done in many ways—from hacking into third- party vendor's com-puters or hacking into your *own* computer.

Once it's out there, it's hard to stop, but not impos-sible. First, you can call your credit card company and let them know that your credit card information may have been stolen and that you need for them to send you a new card with a new number. Second, you can contact the three major credit agencies—TransUnion, Equifax, and Experian—and have them

keep all your tax papers in one folder—this should include all the forms you receive from your employer, forms issued by the government, and (if you have one) your accountant. In another folder keep all your medical expenses that include your primary care doctor, dentist,

put a lock on your account, so that you would be the only one to be able to unfreeze your account moving forward. This is a vital move, because it will protect you from third parties who may try to use your information to gain access to new credit cards—without you knowing. Or third, you can contact a credit monitoring service such as LifeLock, PrivacyGuard, or Aura. For a range of monthly or yearly fees, they will provide various levels of protection.

Unfortunately, most people only become aware of identity theft *after* it has occurred. While it is difficult to stop, it is always a good idea to make sure all your credit purchases and bills are yours. As you go through your monthly credit card statement, make it a point to see if you recognize all the purchases listed as your own. Obviously, low vision may slow down the process, but it's important to keep on top of it.

hospital bills, health insurance, and prescription costs. In yet another folder, keep any receipts you received with payments. If you run a business, you can keep all that financial information in another separate folder. Remember, colored folders can help.

PREPARING YOUR OWN TAX RETURNS

The first thing to know is that, if you are going to prepare your own taxes, nearly all the tax forms you are required to fill out are available in large-print formats. Tax regulations can be very complex, so don't hesitate to ask for help from someone who can help you. Some people are very good at this, however, if you do not understand what you owe and what deductions you can take, join the club. You will probably need to hire someone to complete your tax forms for you. You don't want to pay more than is required, and you need to make your payments by the deadlines.

WORKING WITH AN ACCOUNTANT

All accountants are not the same. If you do not have an accountant, ask your friends, relatives, or business associates for recommendations. Once you have some names of accountants, go online to read any reviews that are posted regarding their work. If necessary, find an accountant who has worked with people who qualify for visual impairment and/or medical deductions. If you have not kept your financial papers in order, ask if the accountant has a person who can help you put all your papers together before he or she sits down with you. The fact is, hiring a professional accountant may save you time and money in the long run.

TAX DEDUCTIONS
FOR THE VISUALLY IMPAIRED

In order to qualify for such tax deductions, your doctor should provide you with paperwork and documentation that states you are legally blind under the guidelines of the state you live in. You then take this documentation to your local social services department of the Social Security Administration. As you will read below, this may entitle you to special benefits and services.

■ Like any taxpayer you are eligible for the standard deduction. If you are blind, you may also be eligible for a special deduction. The amount depends on the tax year and whether you are single, married, or have dependents.

■ If you are employed and require special visual devices to do your work, costs to you may be deductible. Be sure to keep all your receipts to give to your tax person.

TRUST ME!

Beware. According to recent FBI statistics, Americans over the age of 60 lost over $3.4 billion to financial fraud and most of them had normal vision! Strongly resist the urge to follow the advice of someone who tells you, "I can double your money in six months. Just trust me." If it sounds too good to be true it probably is and may be a scam. The number of scams in today's world is at an all-time high, and they often affect the lives of very smart, sighted people. Even if the scheme comes from a relative, think twice! No, maybe think three times. Ask an expert if the plan makes sense, and what your potential risks are.

Also beware of telephone scam artists who prey on older folks to steal their money. If someone calls and whispers, "Hey, Grandma, this is your grandson and I'm in a bind and need your help. Please send me $2,000 dollars, and here's how" you should hang up. All you have to do iso check with other family members to learn what the real status of your grandson is. These smooth talkers can really sound convincing, especially using Artificial Intelligence to create similar-sounding voices of people you may know!

■ Like other taxpayers, your medical expenses are deductible if they reach a certain amount. Keep these receipts, too. This includes transportation expenses incurred when going to appointments to doctors, dentists, pharmacies, and physical therapy centers.

Work with your tax preparer to address all these points. Try to keep the same person from one year to another so he or she will understand your financial and visual needs at any given point in time.

GROWING YOUR MONEY

Some of us are very conservative with the way we invest our money, while others tend to feel comfortable taking some risks. The impact of having low vision may play a role in how and where we invest our money. Much of this depends on how much money we have to invest. Depending upon your current worth, your expenses, and your future needs, you may want to invest enough to maintain your current lifestyle— given a few of the changes we have already discussed in this book.

There are a number of places you may choose to place your money—a bank, a certificate of deposit (CD), the stock market, bonds, or a real estate investment trust (REIT) to mention just a few. Each has its own pluses and minuses.

If you choose to put your money in any such investments, it is wise to check with someone who knows the area. It can be a bank manager, a stockbroker, and/or a financial planner. It's important to determine your level of risk, the need for current income, your tax situation, and what would be best for you. Ask your friends what company was safe and reliable for them.

If you are working with an investment advisor, ask if you can get your reports in large-print formats, audio, or in braille.

JOB OPPORTUNITIES

You may be surprised by the many opportunities for persons with low vision or blindness to work in today's marketplace. Experts point out that your vision does not determine your intelligence, skill level, or willingness to work. Today, both large and small corporations recognize the talents and skills of many people with vision impairments who just need special visual equipment known as "assistive technology" to do their jobs.

Many people with low or no vision hold down successful, well-paying jobs when provided with devices to compensate for their visual loss. In fact, the Americans with Disabilities Act (ADA) *requires* employers to provide *reasonable* accommodations for those who have low vision or blindness. But you, the employee, must first make the employer aware of your specific limitations and the tools needed for you to perform your job.

Depending upon a person's skills, talents, and education, those with vision loss may hold any number of jobs:

■ Professional careers such as lawyer, architect, and even doctors and other medical personnel.

■ Other professions include teachers, college professors, guidance counselors, and even librarians—and that's just for starters.

■ Business careers are also available as financial analyst, marketing experts, and human resource manager.

These are just some of the careers possible for those with vision loss, largely because of recent technological breakthroughs.

You may be thinking you would like to have a job similar to one of those listed above, but you don't have the training, education, or financial resources to achieve that goal. Not to worry, there are organizations that provide scholarships for low-vision or blind students of any age. For example, the American Council of the Blind (ACB) partners with other organizations, businesses, and individuals to offer scholarships for undergraduates, graduate students, and students attending technical colleges. (See Chapter 12, *Jobs, Careers & Employment*, page 216 and *Resources*, page 313 for more information about scholarships.)

FEDERAL STUDENT AID

The U.S. Department of Education offers the Federal Student Aid program to help students who are visually impaired or blind to pay for further schooling beyond high school.

There are many other organizations offering scholarships for you. (See *Resources*, page 315.) Keep in mind that today there are many online colleges, universities, and trade schools that offer classes and degrees in all kinds of fields. There are also scholarships available to assist and help you pay for visual resources necessary to see or read aloud your textbooks. You could work from home without the stress of campus life and earn your desired degree. Or if you would like the experience of going to school and even living on campus there are resources for that too.

If you need help with your job search, there are a number of organizations specifically designed to provide career information, training, and job placement. (See Chapter 12, *Jobs, Careers, & Employment*, page 216 and *Resources*, page 313.)

FINANCIAL ASSISTANCE

If a job is not an option for you and if you have low vision or are blind, there are many resources to help you both financially and in other ways depending on your income and resources. These include governmental support, private foundations, and local agencies. Let's start with government programs.

They offer everything from guidance and support to financial relief and education for all ages.

FEDERAL AND STATE SUPPORT

Federal, state, and local governments recognize the difficulty of making ends meet when you have low vision or blindness. You can't drive yourself to and from job interviews and, of course, your job opportunities seem limited. Therefore, they offer several programs to assist you.

Internal Revenue Service (IRS) ABLE Accounts

Under the IRS code of the 420(a) section, the IRS allows states to administer a savings account called the Achieving a Better Life Experience Account, better known as an ABLE Account. These accounts are designed to help people with physical disabilities. Just like an IRA account, the ABLE account allows you to put money into it for investing without having to pay state or federal taxes on the additional interest made in it. Also there are no taxes or penalties on withdrawals from this account as long as the money is used to pay qualified disability expenses. The maximum amount of money to deposit in an ABLE account is currently $18,000 annually.

All states, except for Wisconsin, manage their state ABLE accounts. To open an account, you contact your own state's ABLE program by phone or online. (See *Resources*, page 300.)

Medicare and Medicaid

Medicare is a federal program that offers health insurance for people who are 65 years or older. Medicaid is both a federal and state program based upon a limited income. Both programs pay for a wide range of medical services. If you have both Medicare and Medicaid and are visually impaired you should qualify for better healthcare coverage, lower out-of-pocket costs, and vision and dental care. You may also qualify for long-term care, home healthcare, and prescription drug coverage.

You are also eligible for monthly help with everyday needs. These include a monthly credit to buy healthy groceries, over-the-counter products, and help to pay utilities such as electricity, gas, water, and internet service. (See *Resources*, page 307.)

National Deaf-Blind Equipment Distribution Program

National Deaf-Blind Equipment Distribution Program, which is also called *I Can Connect* program, is a federal and state program that provides free equipment and training for those with both significant hearing and vision loss who meet federal income guidelines. It is funded by the Federal Communications Commission (FCC). The program provides a variety of tech devices such as smartphones, tablets, computers, braille devices, and more. It is administered by the state where you reside. To apply, go to the ICanConnect website. (See *Resources*, page 323.)

Social Security Disability Benefits

If you have low vision or blindness and are completely unable to work or perhaps can only be partially employed, you may be eligible for benefits from Social Security. To qualify, your vision cannot be corrected by lenses, medication, or surgery. To help you complete the necessary Social Security application forms, they are available in braille and in audio CD format.

There are two types of Social Security benefits that may be available for you: Social Security Disability Insurance (SSDI) and Supplemental Security Income (SSI).

Social Security Disability Insurance (SSDI)

SSDI benefits depend on your work history and the amount of Social Security taxes—called *credits*—you have paid in past years. You may also qualify if your parents or spouse have paid Social Security taxes, also called *credits*. Monthly benefits cover medical care, living expenses, and even rent or a mortgage. The size of monthly payments you would receive depends on the state where you reside.

Supplemental Security Income (SSI)

A second Social Security program is Supplemental Security Income (SSI), which is based on need. If you have limited or no income and few resources, you may qualify for monthly SSI payments. Under this program you may also qualify for Supplemental Nutrition Assistance Program (SNAP) to pay for food and state benefits like Medicaid to cover medical costs.

To qualify for either SSDI or SSI, you must have a report from your eye doctor about your vision and the most recent results of a vision test. You also need to provide information about your income, resources, and living arrangements. You can apply online, by phone, or in person at your local Social Security office. (See *Resources,* page 311.)

NATIONAL FOUNDATIONS

There are also non-governmental organizations that may have resources for you. For example, the National Federation of the Blind (NFB) is such an agency that supports low-vision and blind persons.

American Council of the Blind

This organization advocates on issues related to civil rights, educational opportunities, vocational training, Social Security benefits, and health and social services on behalf of people with visual impairments. (See *Resources*, page 300–301.)

Family Caregiver Alliance

This organization's mission is to improve the lives of family caregivers and those people for whom said care is given. They provide state leads to find those public, nonprofit, and private programs and services located closest to the family. These resources include government health and disability programs, legal resources, disease-specific organizations, and more—all designed to help the family cope with the care of a disabled individual. (See *Resources*, page 305.)

National Federation of the Blind (NFB)

This organization offers various resources to its

members and the public. The NFB provides access to assistive devices, computer technology, and publications that enhance the lives of people with vision loss. Assistive devices include a Free White Cane program that has donated almost 100,000 white canes to blind persons since 2008. Publications include magazines, newsletters, and books on topics of interest to the low-vision community such as blindness, advocacy, education, and employment. (See *Resources*, page 308.)

National Industries for the Blind

The National Industries for the Blind (NIB) works with other agencies to enhance opportunities for personal and economic independence to those people who are blind by creating employment opportunities. In addition, they offer career training to provide people with the skills required for manufacturing and professional services careers. (See *Resources*, page 314.)

NoisyVision

This non-profit provides a compiled list of Facebook groups designed to support people who are blind and visually impaired. They also produce videos, publish prose, and promote visual arts and artistic events. In addition, they organize trips to increase the mobility potential of those with visual impairments. (See *Resources*, page 308.)

LOCAL PROGRAMS

Your community may also have resources and programs to assist you. You could call your Chamber of Commerce to ask for sources to provide you with local help. Two such services in many communities are the *Lions Club International* and *Meals on Wheels*.

Lions Club International

This international organization provides resources and financial help to people with visual impairments. It often provides assistance in home adaptation needs. In order to learn what services may be available in your community, you must connect with the local chapter nearest you. (See *Resources*, page 306.)

Now you know about several government agencies and private foundations that can help you with supplemental income, free vision devices, training, and so much more. A relative or friend with normal vision can help you investigate these and apply for these opportunities. These programs could change your life and help make things a lot easier.

Meals on Wheels America

Meals on Wheels America is a nationwide volunteer organization present in virtually every community in America that delivers daily delicious, nutritious meals to persons over 60 years of age *or* those who are disabled *or* those who are housebound and unable to provide nutritious meals for themselves. Although Meals on Wheels is a national organization, each community sets up its own program. Unfortunately, there may be a waiting list in your community.

You may qualify for this service, which is either free or priced at a very low cost. A recommended contribution of $1.80 USD per day is suggested but not required and many receive meals at no cost. No eligible person is denied. Certainly, if you can contribute more that would be much appreciated because the organization depends on donations alone.

A central kitchen prepares healthy, simple meals which are then delivered to your home by volunteers. Your spouse or caregiver can also receive a meal. This volunteer can also check to see you are okay. This service is a potential blessing to you and your family, who would be delighted to know that you are getting regular meals and that someone is checking on you. To find a Meals on Wheels in your community, go online to Meals on Wheels America and enter your zip code. (See *Resources*, page 307.)

CONCLUSION

The goal of this chapter is to help you with the task of managing your personal finances, finding a job if desired, funding to support further education, and/or obtaining financial help if necessary. Low vision and blindness can greatly affect the goals and aspirations of any person, but that doesn't mean that the hopes of living a full and rewarding life cannot be achieved. It takes patience and persistence, but it can be done. Hopefully, the information in this chapter can provide you with a few pathways to securing a brighter future.

10

Health Matters

Low vision or blindness can have a major impact when it comes to the matters of your health—and it isn't just about your vision. The effect of vision loss can affect every aspect of your life—from your physical and psychological well-being to your ability to monitor the medications you may be taking. It is important to recognize and understand the many health-related issues that may come with significant vision loss—and what solutions there may be to handle each one.

We are all different in the way we live our everyday lives. However, there are a number of common factors that can and will affect the state of our health. If we don't pay attention to them, it's likely we will pay the consequences. In this chapter, we will discuss the most common health-related problems related to low vision. This will include your psychological issues, your diet and exercise activities, your medical supervision, and your handling of medications. We will also touch on your medical insurance.

THE PSYCHOLOGICAL IMPACT OF LOW VISION

If you have low vision you are more likely to feel lonely, fearful, anxious, depressed, and even angry. It can also become a daily source of frustration. This is not surprising when you think about it.

Losing your vision can be a devastating loss of independence, companionship, and your life's work—all the activities you used to enjoy that depended on your vision, and your place in your family and community. It can bring on many negative feelings that can be overwhelming. Let's talk about each of these problems and consider what can be done to improve them.

LONELINESS AND ISOLATION

No doubt, you no longer can jump in the car, go to the store, visit friends, or go out to eat. It's no wonder that you may feel lonely and isolated. Unfortunately, these are common emotions shared by many people with low vision, especially for those who live alone. If you are experiencing these feelings, you should know that there are things you can do to bring more people into your world by engaging in actions such as the following:

■ Hire a helper to aid you with daily activities—someone who is nice and fun to have around, and who can become a companion and good friend.

■ Go for walks to meet and chat with your neighbors.

■ Join a community group or place of worship. Find out how you can get to meeting places, and/or ask for phone numbers of other members who would love to have a "phone" friend.

■ Find ways to help others. In helping others, you will find you will benefit too!

■ Join a gym and perhaps a class for people who have disabilities who want to exercise.

■ Engage in community activities like picnics, band concerts, plays, and so on.

In other words, get out of your house as often as you can and be with people. Your loneliness will improve, but you may have to take the first steps.

ANXIETY

Anxiety is a normal response to fearful events or perceived fearful threats. Our bodies respond with the secretion of all kinds of chemicals and hormones to confront a real or imagined danger. These chemicals help us to swing into action but the effects they create also make us feel nervous and upset.

Chronic anxiety is a common problem for those with low vision. Not being able to see your world clearly makes you feel fearful about potential threats you can't see. In Chapters 3 and 4, we addressed ways to feel safer in your home, how to prepare for medical and other emergencies, and other steps to take to reduce those anxious feelings.

If this remains a major problem for you, talk to your doctor. A mild tranquilizer may calm your frazzled nerves and make you feel calm and relaxed. But you have to share this information with your doctor to get help.

DEPRESSION

Someone who is depressed has a profound feeling of sadness and may lose interest in doing things. Now, we all have times in our lives when we feel "down," but eventually we perk up and go on. However, someone with low vision may feel depressed a lot more of the time. Loss of vision itself may be a trigger for depression. Other stressful life events can also trigger depression such as the loss of a job, a beloved partner, a close friend, or even a favorite pet.

What is important to know and recognize is that there is help available. Just talking with a trained therapist can be helpful. Tell your doctor how you are feeling emotionally and enlist his or her help. Your doctor can recommend a psychologist, social worker, or psychiatrist who has helped other patients like you.

Taking a prescribed medication like an antidepressant could help greatly. There are many different types of antidepressants your doctor can recommend, so if one doesn't help, we encourage you to ask for a different kind. The right one can make a huge difference in how you feel and cope.

FRUSTRATION

As your sight diminishes, you begin to learn that the many things you did regularly at home with no problems become more difficult to do. You begin to make mistakes having to do things over and over. You buy a device to help you perform a task, and it doesn't work the way you thought. Or you have a new program installed in your smartphone or computer, and it doesn't work right. You try your best to figure out how to use it—and as hard as you try, it just doesn't work. That is very frustrating, and that is unfortunately an all too common occurrence.

Also, keep in mind that as many as two-thirds of the sighted population are *not* tech-savvy. So someone, who is not talented in adapting to new tech devices and has low vision, is going to struggle and experience great frustration. If this describes you, then accept who you are and why you are frustrated—but keep persevering because learning how to use various tech devices could improve your life immeasurably.

The fact is that frustration happens all-too-often to people with low vision, and the answer is—you will need patience. Take a few deep breaths, and relax. Try making that damn thing work a few more times, and if it still refuses to operate correctly, call in a tech or a friend who might help. Sometimes you simply have to laugh it off, and accept the fact that it's going to happen more than once. It's important to understand that frustration can turn into depression, anxiety, and anger, if you let it.

ANGER

Getting angry at what is happening to you can stem from any of the emotions we have already discussed. It can do damage to your heart, arteries, and muscles. It can lead to digestive problems and abdominal pain. It can affect your judgment, and it can chase away the people closest to you. And, as with all the other emotions we have covered, anger is not an easy thing to deal with, but it cannot be ignored.

Should you see this happening to you, go talk to your doctor about what healthy alternatives might be in place to help you deal with this problem. What you don't want is to let these negative feelings build up inside of you, and do nothing about them.

By accepting your situation and making sure you are taking steps to deal with each of these feelings, you can, to a great degree, control the person you are. But there are more things that you can do to gain back that control. As you will learn next, your lifestyle can play an important role in controlling these issues, and more. Eating healthy foods, exercising, and sleeping well can all help your brain cope better with the events in your life.

HEALTHY LIFESTYLE

We hear the term *healthy lifestyle*, but what does that actually mean? Basically, it is the way each of us conducts our daily lives in behaviors that should hopefully promote good health. This includes several components such as eating a healthy diet, engaging in exercise, getting good quality sleep, having some fun each day, and reducing stress in your life. The question is, have you followed a healthy lifestyle before the low vision set in, and if not, can you do so now?

Let's consider the following: Before your vision loss, were you overweight? Were you eating the right foods? Did you actually participate in any regular exercise program, and were you getting enough sleep? Unfortunately, for many of us, we know leading a healthy lifestyle was not a priority. Now that things have changed, it should be a top priority.

■ **Our diets.** So, what's the problem? If you are lucky enough to have meals prepared for you, all you have to do is make sure your meals are well-balanced. Sometimes that means having a discussion with the person doing the cooking about making sure your meals are nutritiously balanced. On the other hand, if you are in charge of making your own meals, it can be a bit more challenging. The process of shopping, preparing foods, cooking, and cleaning up is not any easier with low vision.

For some people, it's a lot easier to order in, if the cost isn't a problem. For others, opting to stick with the same basic dishes every day makes sense. Sometimes it's easier to just have a box of snacks nearby. The question is, are you getting the right nutrition to maintain your body's needs and a healthy body weight?

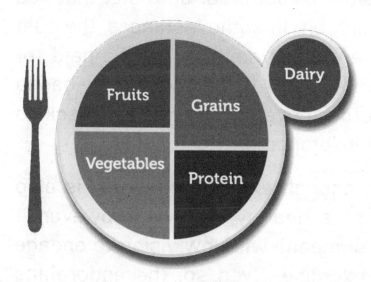

This USDA illustration shows four different food groups and their percentages on your plate. Also recommended is an 8-ounce beverage at every meal.

Your doctor may have suggested, "You need to eat a healthy diet!" But what does that mean? To encourage all Americans to eat better, the government has published the following figure to show the types of foods and their proportions in every meal.

So, every meal should contain fruits, vegetables, grains, protein foods, and a beverage such as milk, water, tea, or coffee but not soda and other sugary drinks. Consuming beverages between meals is important too, so you don't become dehydrated. Even with all that said, bad food habits are hard to break. As we have discussed, the psychological impact of low vision can increase the desire to eat the wrong foods that much more.

Don't be afraid to contact a food nutritionist who can help you plan a realistic diet for weight loss or for better nutritional value—or both. Set up a diet that you feel comfortable being on. In some instances, the cost of working with a registered dietitian can be paid for by a medical insurance plan if the problem is based on diabetes or another covered condition. (Check to see if your medical insurance provides coverage.)

■ **Exercise.** Getting enough exercise each day is also another vital part of a healthy lifestyle. However, it can be difficult for someone with low vision to engage in most forms of exercise. Even so, the endorphins it creates in your brain can make you feel better—and can also help you work off those extra calories. Despite your vision loss, here are a few strategies and exercises that may work for you.

■ **Join a gym.** If you have a sighted friend who likes to workout at a gym, tag along to see what exercises you can do there together. Start slow with any new exercise. Often, there is a track to walk around. You could walk together, perhaps touching her or his arm to stay within the lanes.

There will also be various types of exercise equipment, from treadmills to bicycles to StairMasters to barbells, to increase your strength and endurance. Here, too, work with a buddy nearby, until you feel comfortable enough to work on the equipment alone.

If the gym has a swimming pool, there may be opportunities to walk or swim within lanes or even to join a water aerobics class. A gym membership doesn't have to be expensive. There are many gyms that offer low competitive membership fees and low-cost classes. You should also consider going to a YMCA (Young Men's Christian Association) or YWCA (Young Women's Christian Association), which can be found throughout the country.

■ **Walking.** Walking is a good source of exercise; however, it can be tricky for low-vision folks. If you have a treadmill at home and feel safe using it, make sure you always attach the safety cord that stops the machine in case you fall. If you are unable to see the settings, make sure to keep a lighted magnifying glass nearby.

You can also ask Alexa to set a time to let you know how long you have been on the machine. You can also ask her to play your favorite music. If you don't have Alexa, you can set a time to let you know when to stop and play music on your smartphone. However you set up your treadmill walk, try to gradually increase the time you walk each day. Try aiming for at least a half-hour or more per day.

Walking outdoors is where things get a little more complicated. If your neighborhood has uneven or cracked sidewalks, you might need to walk with a friend to help you avoid these all-too-common hazards. You might also consider mapping out a walking path that avoids most of these potential pitfalls. If the weather is rainy, snowy, or icy, and you don't have a treadmill, you could walk inside depending upon the design and size of your home. Or you could ask a friend to walk with you in a nice indoor shopping mall.

■ **Exercise bike.** An exercise bike may be safer than a treadmill because the risk of falling is less. Again, if you can't see the settings, try using a magnifier. You can ask Alexa to time your bike ride and you can play music while doing so. You can also watch TV, listen to a podcast, or play music on your radio, all while you are biking.

■ **Dancing.** Moving your body to music is another way to go. Choose a space in your house where you won't bump into furniture or trip on anything. Choose whatever music you love and move in time to the rhythm. The intensity of the exercise could range from just rocking back and forth, to moving with speed in your space. Add arm movements for extra benefits. Have fun!

■ **Ideal weight**. Part of a healthy lifestyle is maintaining a healthy weight. If you struggle with your weight, you have lots of company—especially among those with low vision. The reasons are simple—you reach for high-calorie foods that require no preparation, taste good, and make you happy. Also, exercising to shed all those excess calories is difficult. Ask your doctor to help you set goals and perhaps refer you to a nutritionist who can help you set up a reasonable program.

■ **Sleep.** Getting enough high-quality sleep is also vital for good health. After all, only during deep sleep does your brain do "housekeeping chores" to get rid of wastes that your brain accumulated the previous day. If you are sleep-deprived, you probably wake up feeling tired, grumpy, and depressed. For the visually impaired, sleep problems are common. The reasons are lack of sunlight exposure (which sets your sleep cycle,) lack of exercise, and perhaps foods and beverages loaded with caffeine. (See the inset below for more tips on getting a good night's sleep.)

WAYS TO PROMOTE GOOD SLEEP

Many people have a hard time falling asleep. There are a number of proven things you can do to get the sleep you need, including the following:

■ **Set a bedtime.** Choose a time that will give you seven to eight hours of sleep, or whatever you need to feel well-rested. Try to maintain that bedtime every night so your body and brain get used to the routine. Keep in mind that if you experience daytime sleepiness, this could be due to not getting enough good quality sleep at night.

■ **Naps.** If you nap too much in the daytime, you probably will have trouble at night so resist the urge to sleep during the day. However, if you feel better having a brief nap each day and sleep well at night, then keep that routine.

■ **Bedtime routine.** Have a set bedtime routine where you begin to unwind and relax from the day. Stop texting and answering your phone. Avoid alcohol in the evening. While it may make you feel sleepy at first, you may wake up in the middle of the night and be unable to go back to sleep. A cup of chamomile tea or warm milk along with a light snack of whole grain crackers with peanut or almond butter, or a bowl of low-sweetened cereal may help you relax. Protein foods promote sleep, while excessively sugary foods are stimulating.

Do exercises earlier in the day, not in the evening. Take a warm bath or shower. Play quiet, relaxing music. Or ask Alexa or your smartphone to read from a book that is not too stimulating.

■ **Bedroom.** Use your bed and bedroom for sleep only. Watch TV or use your smartphone and computer elsewhere. At night keep the temperature cool, but not cold. Keep it dark, but have lights you can easily turn on, if you need to get up.

An Alexa or similar device in your bedroom can turn on smart plugs and lights if asked. It can also tell you the time and set a wake-up alarm. If you have trouble sleeping, it can play the sound of soft rain on the roof or waves at the seashore or quiet, calming music. In the morning, you can even ask it what the weather forecast is.

■ **No caffeine.** Try to avoid caffeinated foods and beverages such as coffee, tea, and chocolate after 6 pm; some people get to sleep better if they stop ingesting caffeine earlier on during the day.

If you still experience problems sleeping, consider taking a natural supplement such as melatonin or a magnesium tablet. And if they don't work, talk to your doctor about taking something stronger. Getting a good night's sleep is that important.

■ **Have fun.** Adding fun and enjoyment to your life will also improve your health. In Chapter 6 (which covers *Entertainment*), we discussed many ways to have fun and bring joy and happiness to you. Find ways each day to enjoy and appreciate life.

■ **Reduce stress**. In today's world, too much stress is a daily problem for most of us. Reducing this amount leads to a healthier lifestyle. First, identify those things in your life that stress you out. Are there ways to reduce these factors? For example, if listening to the news fills you with anxiety, find something else to watch or listen to instead. Or if a certain relative or friend drives you nuts, consider if you should reduce the frequency of those visits or conversations.

Eating well, exercising, and getting enough sleep

will all help you reduce your stress. Ask your doctor if there are Tai Chi or Yoga classes in your community, and if they include instruction for vision-impaired students. These are great forms of stress-relieving exercise to build and maintain muscle tone, improve balance and flexibility, and help you relax.

There you have it—many ways to improve your lifestyle. While these lifestyle improvements will generally improve your health and make you feel better, they unfortunately won't improve your vision or stop its decline.

HOME MEDICAL DEVICES

For years, people with low vision and blindness were dependent on others to help them take their temperature, blood pressure, blood sugar levels, and so much more. With the miracles of technology, there are home medical devices available that can not only provide a person with accurate test readings but also tell them verbally what the results are. These include thermometers, pulse and oxygen monitors (pulsimeters), blood pressure cuffs, and weight scales. (We will learn more about what's available in Chapter 17, *Medical Devices*, page 285.)

These new devices allow a person the freedom to test themselves. Consider the case of proliferative diabetic retinopathy (PDR), a disease that requires several blood tests to be taken every day. For those with low vision resulting from PDR, it was a difficult or impossible procedure to do without the help of a sighted person. Today, things have changed greatly. (See inset on page 181 regarding PDR.)

Unfortunately, there are still a number of health issues that require home monitoring, but there are no devices that allow you to monitor yourself. However, with the development of Artificial Intelligence (AI) combined with technological advancements, new systems may be on the drawing boards. It is important then to keep asking your doctors about any new devices that might improve your own ability to monitor yourself.

DEALING WITH POOR BALANCE AND WEAKNESS

For some people, low vision brings on problems with balance, instability, falling, weakness, and/or dizziness. These are all issues that can greatly limit your ability to move from one place to another. If you find yourself having these issues, there are two treatments that can help overcome these issues. The first is physical therapy (PT), and the second is occupational therapy (OT).

PHYSICAL THERAPY (PT)

Physical therapy, sometimes called *physiotherapy*, uses special exercises and devices to restore problems with standing, walking, or balance. You may be surprised by how the right PT can improve your balance and stability and help you find exercises suitable for you after just a few sessions.

PROLIFERATIVE DIABETIC RETINOPATHY (PDR)

Proliferative diabetic retinopathy is a chronic condition that can cause progressive damage to the retina, which leads to vision loss and blindness. It is caused by high blood sugar (glucose) and is therefore linked directly to diabetes.

For those with PDR, it is important to check and record their blood sugar level several times a day. Patients would measure their blood sugar levels by pricking their finger with a small needle to produce a blood drop. The drop would then be placed on a test strip in a glucose meter, and the meter would show the blood sugar level. For people with low vision resulting from PDR, it was not an easy procedure to do, in many cases, without the help of a sighted person.

Better options are now available. While a talking glucose meter for low vision and blindness called

Prodigy Voice Talking Glucose Meter tells a person their glucose level, it still requires use of a finger prick. However, modern technology has come to the rescue with a way for people to continuously know their glucose level without finger pricks or the use of one's eyes.

Dexcom G6 and *FreeStyle Libre 3* are glucose monitoring systems (GMS) that help any diabetic know immediately what their blood sugar is, including those with visual impairment. There is a glucose sensor that is attached to the upper arm or abdomen by someone with sight. Diabetics report that this is painless. This sensor reads their glucose level and sends the result to a smartphone warning them when their blood sugar is too high or too low. Apple iPhones and many Android devices are compatible with these devices. (See Chapter 17, *Medical Devices*, page 285.)

If you are suffering from PDR, ask your tech person or pharmacist if your smartphone is compatible with such a monitoring system prescribed by your doctor. Medicare and private insurers should pay for the device. If you have Medicaid, many states, but not all, will cover the cost. Your doctor's nurse or your pharmacist can show you how to use the unit.

OCCUPATIONAL THERAPY (OT)

Occupational therapy is designed to help a patient regain his ability to perform normal everyday activities. OT helps patients perform activities related to daily living. Such activities include basic self-care tasks as handling transportation, shopping, preparing meals, putting away groceries, using a computer, managing medications, doing laundry, housework, and basic home maintenance.

In some cases, physical therapists or occupational therapists can come to your home if you are unable to go to them. One advantage of this is that the therapist will personally see your house, determine how to address problems, and help you use your space to exercise. If you need this type of care, ask your doctor to recommend the name of a physical therapist or occupational therapist. Private health insurance, Medicare, and Medicaid cover the costs of PT and OT. However, the extent of Medicaid benefits will depend on the state where you live.

YOUR DOCTORS

As you have read above, maintaining a healthy lifestyle is important for good health. Also important is getting routine medical and dental check-ups so that potential

health issues are identified and treated early. Establishing a good relationship with your doctors, dentist,
and pharmacist is an important first step. First, let's
discuss types of doctors you may have.

PRIMARY CARE DOCTOR

Finding a primary care doctor who you know and trust
is important. Establishing ways to communicate with
her/him, the nurse or nurse practitioner, and others on
the office staff, including the person who answers the
phone, is critical. They each need to understand your
vision problems, what you can and cannot see, and
the best ways to communicate with you.

For example, if they plan to post information for
you on a website like MyChart (or other systems
where you can access your medical records), this may
not be helpful unless you have a way to enlarge the
site on your smartphone or computer so the results
can be read aloud. Even then it may be difficult to
navigate the site in order to find messages from your
healthcare staff, to message them back, to see your
lab tests, or to schedule appointments.

Also, it is common for doctors to print out a summary of your office visit that contains your vital signs,
the diagnosis, dietary and exercise advice, prescription drugs, and follow-up appointment. You could ask
them to enlarge the print. You could then use a hand

magnifier or an instrument called the OrCam device to read it aloud.

Explain to your doctor the extra help you need due to your vision. It is crucial that they take more time to explain the treatments they may want you to follow—physical therapy, dietary changes, and also your prescription drugs and how and when to take them. If the doctor doesn't seem interested in going the extra mile to help you, then find a doctor who will be!

OPTOMETRIST AND OPHTHALMOLOGIST

What is the difference between an optometrist and ophthalmologist? While they can both diagnose, treat, and manage eye disorders, optometrists tend to provide routine eye care. Ophthalmologists, however, specialize in certain eye disorders and can perform surgery when necessary. As a proactive patient, you may want to keep in close touch with your eye doctor. The doctor may have new drugs, visual devices, or surgical treatments that could significantly help you see better.

For example, there are new drug treatments for both wet and dry macular degeneration that can stabilize your vision or actually improve it in some cases. There are also new drug treatments for diabetic retinopathy. So having regular appointments with both eye doctors will help you keep up on the newest treatments for your eye condition.

CLINICAL TRIALS

You may want to inquire about any new and/or existing clinical trials for your eye problem. A clinical trial
is the standard method used by drug companies to
establish how effective a drug they are developing
truly is. A group of patients with the same disease
are asked to participate in the study. Once the
group is large enough, they are then divided into
two groups. One group is given a new treatment,
while the other receives a *placebo* (a drug that contains no active ingredient and provides no helpful
effect) or no treatment at all. At the end of the trial,
results are compared to see if those patients given
the new treatment have benefited from significantly
better results than those who received either the
placebo—or, in fact, no treatment at all. Clinical trials
are supported by the government through eye health
institutions, and by drug companies that aim to come
up with better and more effective treatments.

Ask your eye doctor if there are any new clinical
trials for your particular eye disease, and whether
or not you would qualify to participate. These trials
are generally conducted in more than one medical
center around the U.S. and the world, so there may
be one close to you. You can also find them online

at the National Eye Institute. You will be carefully screened to determine if you meet the strict criteria for the study in question. (See *Resources*, page 307 for more information.)

If chosen for a clinical trial, you will be fully informed about the procedure, any adverse side effects (if they are aware of any), possible benefits, and your rights and responsibilities as a participant. You will be randomly assigned to receive either the new treatment or a placebo. You will be carefully monitored with free eye care, free transportation to the treatment center, and even a small monetary amount to compensate you for your time. You may not learn which group you have been in until the trial is over.

Why should a clinical trial interest you? One reason to participate is to advance the understanding of your eye disease, which could be of great service both to you and future patients. Another helpful motive for participation is that you would be one of the first to receive a new and potentially beneficial treatment. Be assured that these clinical trials are conducted with great care to ensure no damage occurs. Many scientists and doctors oversee these trials, so you should always be in good hands.

PODIATRISTS

Another doctor to see regularly is a foot doctor or *podiatrist*. You probably struggle to cut your nails, especially your toenails. Good foot care is important if you want to be active. If you are diabetic, it is even more important that infection of your feet and/or toes is prevented or treated early. Ask your doctor to recommend a doctor near you.

DENTISTS

Oral health and dental care are also important for good health. You want teeth that chew your food well, don't hurt, and give you a nice smile. If you have problems with cavities or bleeding gums, discuss with your dentist and dental hygienist how you can better care for your mouth.

Explain your vision limits so you can all work together for a healthier mouth. Ask if an electric toothbrush, an electric toothbrush with a WaterPik (tiny little brushes sometimes referred to as "mini-Christmas trees"), or any other devices they might recommend as helpful. You may not be able to see your teeth, but you should be able to navigate your mouth with your fingers.

Getting good healthcare for your whole body will improve the quality of your life.

TAKING MEDICATIONS

Medications include both over-the-counter (OTC) drugs, vitamins and other supplements, and prescription drugs. Over-the-counter drugs are meds that don't require a prescription to purchase. Neither do supplements. Ask your doctor or pharmacist if one or more of these would be helpful. Ask how you should take them, when, and how much—these are crucial questions to ask because the typed print on the bottle labels is often hard to read. If you need more information, go online, use your smartphone, or ask Alexa, "What are the directions for taking medicine 'X'? What, if any, are the side effects?"

Your doctor should also give you careful information for prescription drugs—how much to take and when, what the drug does, how long it takes to work, what are side effects, if any, and how to contact the doctor's office if you have problems. Your pharmacist can also give you guidance when you are scheduled to take a particular prescription medication.

KEEPING TRACK OF YOUR MEDS

Keeping track of prescription and over-the-counter meds is difficult for many patients, especially if they have multiple meds to take. As a low-vision person, you have several challenges: You can't read the labels on the bottles, you can't see the tablets or capsules to distinguish one from another, you can't accurately measure out a liquid medication, and it's harder for you to keep track of time.

Unfortunately, many pharmacies are not very helpful, and there is no national recommendation or requirement for how best to assist patients with low vision. On top of that, many pharmacies are short of staff, including pharmacists, so they have little time for individual care.

Try to find a pharmacy near you that has a pharmacist who will go the extra mile to help you. Discuss your vision disabilities, your health needs, and work out a plan for you. Ask the pharmacist what days and hours he or she works so you can best contact him or her, if necessary. However, technology is changing the face of the game as you'll read below.

Here are some related tips to help you:

■ Set daily timers on your smartphone or Alexa to remind you when it's time to take meds. You could even say, "Remind me when it's time to take my insulin, blood pressure pill, diuretic—" and so on, especially if there are different times each day when you need to take different meds.

■ If you take several meds, ask someone you trust to put them into a pillbox organizer for the next week or two. These organizers can be purchased at your drug store or online. Some have 3 to 4 compartments where you can place your morning, noon, dinner, and bedtime pills on a daily basis. Or you could use small, colored paper cups. You might consider attaching a small self-adhesive shelf above your sink where you can place your pills. That way, you will spot them easily and as a reminder for you to take them.

■ You can also ask your pharmacist to pre-package the sets of meds you take in pill containers for a week or a month. They will normally charge a fee to provide this service.

■ If you can't read the labels on prescription bottles, ask your pharmacist to print them in large print—and then affix the bigger instructions to larger pill bottles so that they will fit. A few pharmacies can print labels in braille. To keep your bottles straight, you could put one dot on one bottle, then two dots on another, and so on. Then to find a bottle you need, you simply feel for the dots.

■ There is also the ScripTalk Talking Prescription Label digital tool, which can read the information on a pill container aloud by using the ScripTalk Mobile app or a ScripTalk Station Reader. It can tell you the drug name, dosage, warnings, and more. Several drugstores and supermarket chains—including, among others, Walmart, CVS, Sam's Club, Publix, Winn-Dixie, and Wegmans—are now making this helpful aid widely available.

CONCLUSION

Staying healthy when you have low vision or blindness is not always easy. You are likely to run into numerous problems. While you can't make all of them go away, you can resolve many of them with a little patience— and, hopefully, with some of the suggestions provided in this chapter. For the ones that are harder to solve, don't be afraid to ask others for help. With some creativity and a little help from modern-day technology, lots of problems can be taken care of in a variety of ways.

It's also important to keep in mind that when it comes to your own well-being, a good deal of the responsibility falls on your shoulders. Yes, your doctors can offer you advice, but it's up to you to follow their recommendations and do the things that are best for you. Just because your eyes aren't working the way you hoped, that isn't something that should prevent you from being healthy—in mind, body, and spirit.

11

Aids for Those Who Are Blind

While many traditional forms of help—such as braille and mobility aids—have been available to blind individuals for decades, with the breakthroughs of high-tech innovations, a new generation of assistive technology has greatly improved and expanded what a blind person can now do. These new devices and software can provide users with a greatly enhanced level of independence and safety never before available.

It is important to point out that many of the recommendations found in the previous chapters can also apply to those who are blind—these range from safety in the home, educational and vocational goals, to the steps required to access both printed and digital information. These suggestions can greatly improve your life, if you are without sight. In the same way, there is much crossover between aids for blind individuals and individuals with low vision.

In this chapter, we will discuss the traditional aids, the additions to these aids that have been improved by the new electronic devices, and digital programs that have revolutionized assistive technology for the blind.

ORIENTATION AND MOBILITY (O&M) TRAINING

When learning to travel safely and independently, there are two basic hurdles people who are blind must learn to overcome. First is knowing physically where they are in order to get from one location to another. This is called *orientation* to their environment. The second is learning how to travel from point A to point B, referred to as *mobility*. For most with low vision and blindness, these are two important life skills that need to be learned.

Orientation and mobility instructors are specialists who train people with a visual impairment to develop orientation skills and navigate/travel through their environment. O&M training is individualized for each student based upon many factors such as age, physical skills, and goals. O&M teaches a person to know their location (orientation to the environment) and then to create a plan to travel safely to their desired location (mobility).

ORIENTATION

Orientation is a skill to know where one is located in the environment and to know how to plan a route to safely travel to the desired location. A mental map of the route is needed to remain oriented. Knowledge of landmarks and clues along the desired route is extremely important. These enable the traveler to know their location while traveling along any given route.

Today, there are different apps on a smartphone that can provide locations, directions, and landmarks along with their histories. However, to safely reach their destination, other advanced skills are necessary. These skills include crossing streets, taking public transportation, and the ability to use mobility aids such as a long cane, dog guide, and smartphone apps.

MOBILITY

Through O&M training, students are taught how to use mobility aids, such as a white long cane or guide dog, to move safely through their environment. The orientation skills are blended and combined with movement (mobility) through the environment. Orientation and movement are dependent upon each other to provide safe and independent travel. With that in mind, it is important to recognize that each blind person is different and has different skills when it comes to learning how to travel.

Instructors usually conduct training sessions one-to-one. This is done so they can tailor their training to a person's specific skill level, educational and vocational needs, as well as travel goals. O&M lessons typically begin in indoor environments and move progressively to outdoor locations. Other mobility aids may include audio or tactual maps, often combined with the long cane or guide dog. It often will include apps or devices that contain maps for walking and using public transportation.

How Does One Get O&M Training in One's Own City?

The best ways to find out about Orientation and Mobility services in your home area is to contact your state social services department and/or use Google Search to seek out what agencies offer O&M training access.

GUIDE DOGS

There are many guide dog schools in the U.S. and Canada. Potential guide dogs begin their own training as puppies and are taught to socialize. The volunteers who raise the puppies travel with their dogs to many types of social situations including shopping malls, public transportation, concerts, family gatherings, and many more. When the dog is 12 to 15 months old, they begin to receive formal training as a guide dog.

Guide dog schools have a rigorous program that leads to a select few dogs that end up trained to serve the role. The potential blind owner of a dog will most often attend the school for two to four weeks. There, they are matched with a dog that has characteristics needed for the individual. This usually includes the height of the dog, rate of walking speed, and the personality match between the owner and the dog.

Once a match is made, the teaching begins. The lessons are progressive—they begin with indoor travel and eventually move outdoors to residential environments. Later stages will include street crossings, public transportation, and walking in areas with more traffic similar to most downtown environments.

Again, lessons and goals will differ with each individual based upon their skills and physical activity level. Working the guide dog frequently is required, which will allow the dog to retain what he has learned through repetition. Owners should expect to work with their dog daily, or as much as possible, in order for the guide dog to retain the skills he has been taught.

SIGHTED GUIDES

If you have a friend or relative who wishes to help you take walks, accompany you to appointments, or help you go shopping, you can ask them if they would be willing to act as your sighted guide. However, to properly accompany you, it is important that they learn the basics of being a sighted guide in order to be as helpful as possible. There are a number of websites under "sighted guides" that provide important information on how it should be done properly.

There are also a number of volunteer groups located throughout the U.S. and Canada that provide training to volunteers to serve as sighted guides as well. You might contact a national organization to learn if there are any local groups to help find a volunteer to help. (See *Resources*, page 300 for the names of such organizations.)

It is also important for you to take an active role when working with your new sighted guide. There are a number of accompanying techniques that can be used when traveling outside the home. Some of these techniques may provide more reassurance than others/ Explain to the sighted guide how you hope they can help you, and, as they accompany you, which techniques make you feel most comfortable.

LONG WHITE CANES

Most blind people will use a long white cane with a red tip as an aid whenever and wherever they walk. The white and red colors are very bright and easy to see by the public and motorists. The proper use of the long cane is usually taught by an Orientation and Mobility teacher. The method of teaching begins with how to properly hold and use the cane while moving through a variety of environments. The height of the cane should be measured so that it reaches the shoulder of the user. However, some blind users prefer use of an even longer cane

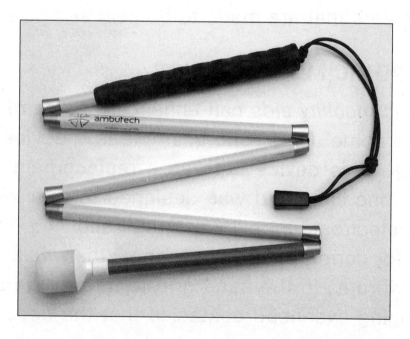

When receiving training from an Orientation and Mobility teacher, the student will usually be trained on the use of a long cane that may be folded when not being used.

The long cane is not a support cane. It is instead a tool intended to reach out in front of the user to locate drop-offs, step-ups, and obstacles from the waist down. The long cane also indicates to the public that the user has a visual impairment. When someone sees a person using a long cane they may decide to offer assistance, which of course can be accepted or rejected by the user. Motorists should be more cautious when they see someone crossing a street using the long cane with bright white and red colors. Most long canes can be folded and used when needed. When not being used, the folding long cane can be stored in a backpack or purse. There are even folding cane holders that are made to be held in a belt.

ELECTRONIC MOBILITY AIDS

Electronic mobility aids can enhance the use of a long cane for some users. One example is a device called WeWALK. This device acts as a replacement handle for any long cane and was designed to turn the cane into an electronic mobility aid—still allowing it to feel natural for normal long cane usage. When walking, this device vibrates in the hand grip to inform the user of low-hanging over-head obstacles that the bottom of a cane will typically miss, such as a sign or tree branch. Users may also upload an app onto their smartphone that allows them to listen to information that

coordinates with the cane to assist them with orientation and public transportation.

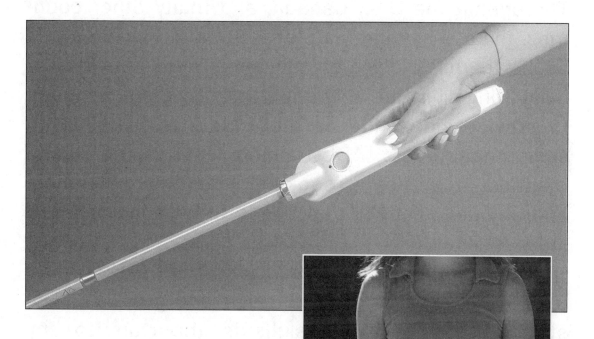

Smart electronic long
canes have detection
technology that alerts you
to over-head obstacles
through haptic and
audible feedback, all
while maintaining the
ground-level feedback
of a standard white
cane. They incorporate
AI technology to help
locate destinations and
navigation information
using voice commands.

ACTIVITIES OF DAILY LIVING (ADL)

Throughout the U.S., Canada, and many other countries, there are programs that teach blind children and adults the basic skills of daily life. These activities of daily living skills are very important. They are designed to provide independence and safety to people with sight impairments. ADL training teaches the fundamentals of self-care, cooking, household cleaning, and any daily activity that needs to be accomplished independently.

The length of these programs varies according to the age, severity of vision loss, and goals of each student. Training these skills is important to any age group. Most of the costs for these services are provided free from a variety of sources. These may include K-12 schools, state-level Vocational Rehabilitation programs, Veterans Administration, and grants that are focused on ADL services.

A major goal is for students to overcome some of their fears and apply what they have learned, so they can become more independent. ADL instruction addresses students' needs on an individualized basis. Each individual has different levels of skills and capabilities. The instructor will individualize an ADL training program for each person. (To learn more about these programs, see *Resources*, page 319.)

BRAILLE (ON PAPER AND REFRESHABLE BRAILLE DEVICES)

Braille is the traditional system of reading and writing for the blind. Named after its inventor, Louis Braille, it has been in use for nearly two hundred years and is devised so that it allows the blind to read by touch. Its letters are composed of raised dots. These dots are formed within units of space known as *braille cells*. Any combination of one to six dots may be raised within each cell, and the number and position of the raised dots within a cell conveys to the reader the letter, word, number, or symbol the cell represents.

There are 64 possible combinations (or characters) of raised dots within a single cell. There are three different grades or versions of braille. These three forms of braille are based upon its use for different languages and/or for specific purposes. (See inset on page 204 regarding braille for details.)

While reading and writing in braille has been a mainstay of education and entertainment for the blind, things are changing rapidly. Today, there are refreshable braille displays with round-tipped pins that rise and lower through holes on its flat surface. This allows the user to read textual output. And just as important, with the advancement in technology, computer programs can now convert written words into spoken words, as we will learn.

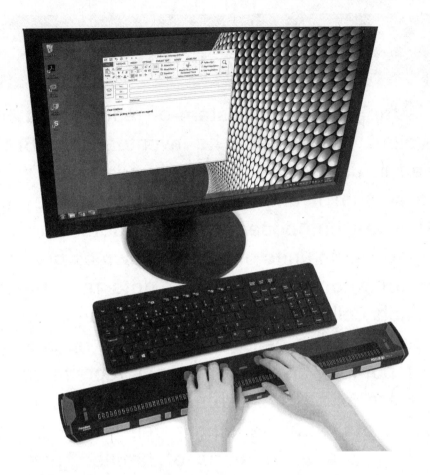

Desktop low-vision machines can be used to read text, labels on cans, and complete puzzles. In addition, users can easily write notes, checks, and complete puzzles.

BRAILLE

Braille is the common writing system used by people who are visually impaired. It has been designed to be used in various languages through the world. To make its use more applicable and convenient, it comes in three forms:

■**Grade 1 braille**. In this form, each possible arrangement of dots within a cell represents only one letter, number, or punctuation sign. Individual cells cannot represent words or abbreviations in this grade of braille. Grade 1 braille is typically used only by those who are just beginning to learn it. As of the early 2000s, a new movement was in place among elementary school teachers of braille to introduce children with sight difficulties to grade 2 braille immediately after teaching the basics of grade 1 braille.

■**Grade 2 braille.** This form was introduced as a space-saving alternative to grade 1 braille. In grade 2 braille, a cell can represent a shortened form of a word. Many cell combinations have been created to represent common words, making this the most popular of the grades of braille. There are part-word contractions, which often stand in for common suffixes or prefixes, and whole-word contractions, in which a single cell represents an entire commonly used word. Words may be abbreviated by using a single letter to represent the entire word, or by using a special symbol to precede either the first or last letter of the word. Books and magazines are produced in grade 2 braille.

■ **Grade 3 braille.** This is essentially a system of braille shorthand. Because it has not been standardized, it is not often used. Instead, it is typically used by individuals for their own personal convenience. It contains over 300 word contractions and makes great use of vowel omission.

If a person is a good braille user, they may use low-tech braille labels to adhere to a variety of objects or locations. A simple low-tech labeler can quickly and inexpensively produce a label with braille characters on it. The label that has a sticky backing can then be placed almost anywhere.

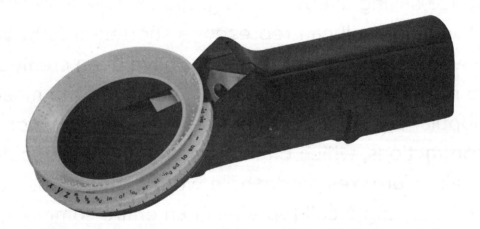

A braille labeler is perfect for a blind person wanting to organize almost anything. This labeler has a tactile dial with braille letters, as well as print letters so a sighted friend can help. The tape has adhesive backing that sticks to what you want to label.

Refreshable Braille Displays

A refreshable braille display is an electromechanical device that displays braille characters and words, usually by means of round-tipped pins raised through holes in a flat surface. Most advanced users today read braille on electronic refreshable devices rather than on braille paper. Braille documents that are printed out on braille paper require huge amounts of paper and space to store the document. Plus, the user needs a braille printer to print the document.

Refreshable braille devices may be connected to a computer or smartphone or they may be used as standalone equipment. The connection may be gotten through Bluetooth or cable systems. Bluetooth is the preferred method for portability. These devices usually range from 18 to 80 braille cells. For users who love braille and are fast and accurate braille readers, refreshable devices are very helpful.

When using electronic braille, the user may also combine it with speech to hear what is being read, or, in some cases, can just turn the speech sound off and depend upon the braille output only. There are several companies that produce these devices—HumanWare, Freedom Scientific, and HIMS are some that are well-known and have been producing these products for many years. (See *Resources,* page 330.)

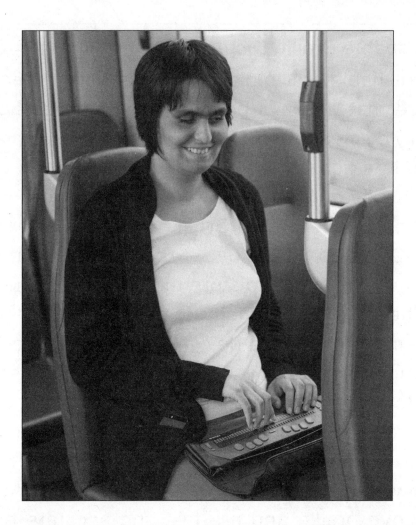

The user using a braille notebook while commuting. The user can create files and content, save files, and later send files to other persons.

MODERN TECHNOLOGIES

In addition to braille, advances in modern technologies have given rise to new and important aids to help the blind read and write. Where reading a printed book was once impossible for people with an advanced visual impairment, today audiobooks are available for everyone. And that's just the tip of an emerging iceberg. Let's explore some of these technological aids that have already begun to change people's lives.

OPTICAL CHARACTER RECOGNITION (SCANNING AND READING)

Optical Character Recognition (OCR) is a technology that transforms printed documents into digital image files. The blind user can take a picture of printed text and then immediately have the text read aloud. The user may also decide to save what has been scanned and then have the document read aloud at a later time. This technology is very important in this information age and provides much independence and opens many doors for employment and professional careers.

There are many varied devices that provide OCR speech output to blind users. Scanning and reading may be part of a desktop or laptop computer. The user may obtain a scanner and appropriate scanning/reading software and connect this to their computer using Bluetooth or cable.

Instead of a computer, a user may prefer to use a device that is a standalone product. These devices are engineered to be very simple to use and portable. With these devices there are few buttons to learn, so that the user can be up and running in no time. An example of this type of product is the Optelec Clear-Reader+, which is a simple standalone scanning and reading device.

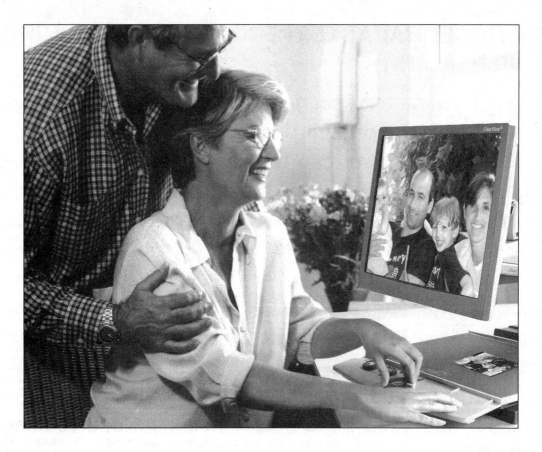

A couple viewing an enlarged family photo with a desktop low-vision machine. These machines can also be used for reading and writing. They feature various brightness levels and modes to see colors or just black and white.

Another way to have scanning and reading capability is to include this technology on a low-vision desktop machine. These machines typically have two cameras (one for live mode when viewing magnified information, and another for taking a picture of the text to be read aloud). The user can use their desktop closed-circuit television (CCTV) to magnify and read as usual, or they have another option where they can take a picture of the text and then have it read aloud to them.

This is great for those persons who require a high degree of magnification and whose eyes become easily fatigued. When fatigue sets in, the user may take a picture of the text and the text is then read aloud. As in all scanning and reading devices, the user can control such things as rate of speech, volume, language, and male or female voices. Shown below is a Topaz OCR desktop machine.

Scanning and reading can be part of a hands-free product that is worn on the user's head. There are several products that have this technology. One example is an Orcam. This product has no low-vision features—it just scans and reads. It can also read text from across the room or signs in an airport, for example.

There are other head-worn devices that have scanning and reading capability, but they also have low-vision features. These devices are much larger than the Orcam, and they provide low-vision magnification as well. (See Chapter 13, *Magnification Options*, page 233 and *Resources*, page 329.)

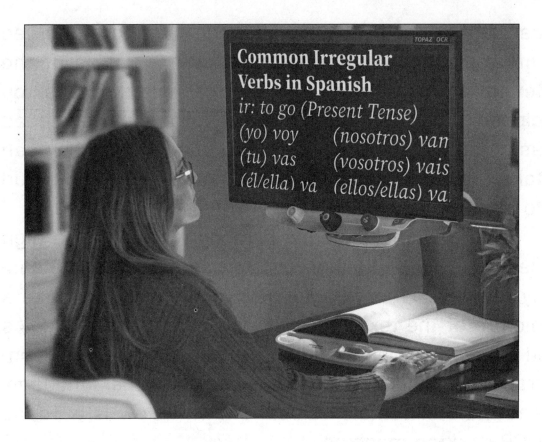

A Topaz desktop low-vision machine, demonstrating how a textbook can be enlarged for easy reading.

SMARTPHONE AND APPS

Blind users can learn how to use standard smart-phones by using the screen-reading software that comes with the phone. VoiceOver screen-reading soft-ware on Apple products—such as the Apple iPhone and *TalkBack* screen-reading software on Android devices—are built into the operating systems of these devices. These speech software utilities allow the user to inter-act with all features of the phone. A learning curve is necessary to learn how to control and use screen-reading software. Using your fingers to swipe and tap on the smartphone screen controls the speech, as well as the desired function on the smartphone. The user can learn these controls with self-paced audio tutorials and/or instruction by teachers.

A SMARTPHONE FOR THE BLIND

Smart Vision 3 is a special smartphone designed for individuals who are blind or severely vision-impaired. Certified by Google, it has a tactile keypad that makes it easier to use. Google Assistant is accessed by pressing a button that lets you place calls, set alarms, and much more. You also have access to Google Play and can order from the Google Play Store. Apps allow you to download Google Gmail, YouTube, and Google Maps, among others.

Apps such as *Seeing AI* have many very helpful functions that include scene, person, and currency identification. Optical character recognition of text is included. This app is very powerful and easy to learn.

The *Be My Eyes* app allows the user to use their smartphone to call a volunteer and then point their smartphone camera toward an object, text, or physical location. The volunteer who is called then tells the user what is being viewed in real time. This service has a modest fee for use. (See *Resources*, page 302.)

COMPUTER ACCESS OPTIONS

For totally blind persons, the options to read information on a computer monitor include speech output (screen-reading) software and a refreshable braille display for those with excellent braille skills. Screen-reading software is very common for blind computer users and has been used since 1980, when home computers began to be used in larger numbers. These software products are continually updated to work well with new operating systems and application software.

Screen-reading software has enabled many people to be successful students and employees. Learning how to use speech software is often done using audio tutorial products, as well as individualized instruction by qualified teachers. A well-known screen-reading software called JAWS (Job Access With Speech) has been produced and continually improved since 1989.

When typing information into a computer, a user who is blind will use a standard keyboard. Learning how to touch-type and learning computer key locations are very important skills to be successful for school and employment. Tactual dots on specific keys can assist in learning the keyboard and where each key is located. Some people may also use voice recognition in combination with touch-typing. Voice recognition uses the computer microphone to replace some of the typing on the keyboard.

Through voice recognition, as we have learned, users can also control one's home environment such as heating and cooling, lighting, and many household appliances. Further, voice-controlled devices allow the user to answer and initiate telephone calls, emails, and text messages.

CONCLUSION

Learning how to travel independently using various mobility aids and public transportation including bus, rail, and car services allows a person to accomplish many goals in their lives. Communication via smartphones and computer software opens the job market for many different types of occupations and careers. For the first time, remote workstations and adaptive computer technology provide many more varied employment opportunities than ever before.

Technology such as OCR and smartphones are very powerful tools. Refreshable braille devices and screen-reading software, along with many handheld portable devices, have opened up many pathways for those without sight. Hopefully, as these technologies continue to evolve, even more breakthroughs will occur—all allowing the blind to live more full and independent lives.

12

Jobs, Careers & Employment

Let's face it. There are a number of jobs that people with low vision or blindness are not going to get. No real openings for airplane pilots or limo drivers, but the fact is there are a good number of positions being filled by people with poor to no vision. There are certainly hurdles to get over, but with the advancements in technology, the opportunities for employment have greatly increased.

Today, people who are visually impaired or blind work in a variety of roles in almost every major category of employment—where vision is not a critical requirement. And as we will learn, the role of the Americans with Disabilities ACT (ADA) of 1990 has opened the door to millions of people whose physical limitations have prevented them from getting hired in the past.

In this chapter, we take a look at the employment statistics dealing with the visually impaired, the government regulations regarding hiring those who are disabled, and we will examine some of the most common barriers faced by those with vision impairments. We will then consider what jobs are out there.

THE STATISTICS

The National Industries for the Blind (NIB) recently did a study on unemployment among people who were blind or visually impaired. The results were not surprising. Of the 3.5 million Americans of working age with visual impairment, 70% were unemployed.

The two major reasons cited for this included public and employer misconceptions about the abilities of people with visual impairment and the hiring managers' perceptions of candidates who are visually impaired or blind. However, we believe there is also a third reason. The psychological impact of losing one's eyesight—whether over time or quickly—can be very traumatic.

People who have worked for years, and counted on their vision to carry out their daily tasks, find themselves suddenly unable to do so. For many, going to work is no longer something they feel capable of doing. Yet, with the right help, this psychological barrier can be overcome. While it may take some time, it *can* be done. (As discussed in Chapter 10, *Heath Matters*, see page 164.)

As the NBI study indicates, the percentage of working men and women with visual impairments is relatively small, but if it was not for the Americans with Disabilities Act (ADA) of 1990, that percentage would likely be even smaller. This act provided protection against discrimination based on disabilities.

THE AMERICANS WITH DISABILITIES ACT (ADA)

Under the ADA, a person with a physical disability must be treated the same way as a person who does not have a disability. In addition, workplaces must accommodate workers' disabilities by providing the things they need to do their jobs. Employers that have 15 or more employees, including state/local governments, employment agencies, and labor unions must provide these people an equal opportunity to benefit from the employment-related opportunities available to others. This includes things like recruitment, hiring, promotions, training, pay, and social activities.

When job applicants or employees request job modifications—that is, changes to the ways things are usually done in an office setting. The disability laws require employers in the private and government sectors to provide reasonable accommodations to their employees and job applicants. Specifically, these modifications must be given to those who have or had an impairment that substantially limits a major life activity—unless doing so would cause undue hardship for the employer. Undue hardship means that the accommodation would be too difficult or too expensive to provide, in light of the employer's size, financial resources, and the needs of the business.

A reasonable accommodation can help a person with a disability apply for a job, perform the duties of a job, or enjoy the benefits and privileges of employment. Some reasonable accommodations include: providing a reader or interpreter for someone who is blind, making a schedule change, installing screen-reading software, providing work at home, allowing leave for disability-related treatment or symptoms, or reassignment to a vacant position where reasonable accommodation is not possible in the current job.

In the past, most companies were not going to alter their office environment to accommodate someone with a disability. However, with the enactment of ADA, people with disabilities now have an equal opportunity to work—not just equal treatment. If you have any questions regarding employment, there are a number of national organizations set up to answer your questions and to help you find a job. You will find the names and contact information for these groups in the *Resources* section of this book. (Under *Resources,* see *Jobs,* page 313, *Scholarships for Careers*, page 315, and *Education for Vocation & Independent Living*, page 315.)

WHAT A WORKSPACE SHOULD HAVE

An accessible physical workspace for blind or visually impaired employees is essential to protect their safety and productivity. Beneficial physical accommodations include the following:

- Accessible meeting room(s)

- Accessible restrooms

- Adjustable lighting

- Clear pathways and unobstructed walkways

- Accessible workstations

- Organized environment

- Tactile raised dots or velcro

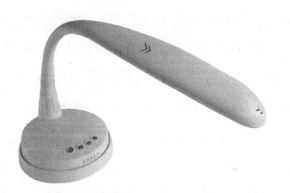 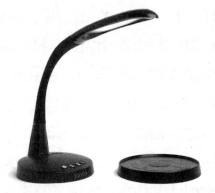

Lamps that focus the light directly on the object or text are very useful and often work best for low-vision users. Features that provide warm and cool light with different levels of brightness are very important.

Technological Support

Assistive technology plays a major role in enhancing the workplace experience for BVI employees. Some of the most effective include:

- Help desk for software support

- Low-vision machines

- Portable low-vision aids

- Refreshable braille displays

- Scanning and text-reading devices

- Screen reader software

- Screen magnification software

- Voice recognition software

Flexible Work Arrangements

Flexible work conditions can greatly benefit individuals with Bilateral Visual Impairment (BVI) by providing the necessary support and accommodations to perform their job duties effectively. These include:

- Flexible work schedules

- Job sharing or part-time work

- Remote work

EMPLOYMENT BARRIERS

There are a number of barriers that make it difficult for visually impaired people to find employment, and in some cases, to hold down a job. These include things like a lack of transportation to the job, the costs involved in purchasing adaptive aids, not having proper vocational training, the negative attitudes of employers, and in some cases, the bad behavior of other employees. There is no doubt that many of these barriers make it difficult to find work, but with a little bit of planning many of them can be overcome. Let's consider some of the most common obstacles.

TRANSPORTATION

Getting from home to a job sounds easy. For most of us, it is relatively simple. You get in your car and drive to work. In a survey by the World Services for the Blind, one hundred percent of participants in their Employment Barriers survey found transportation to work to be a barrier when they are trying to find employment. Oftentimes, those who are visually impaired or blind work in areas where it might be difficult to find public transportation. Employers also may not understand that an employee takes public transportation, and that they may be a few minutes late or early.

Possible Solutions

Even though transportation can be an obstacle, there are possible solutions to consider for each individual. Perhaps consider shared riding programs with other employees, moving near the job site if possible, or obtain orientation and mobility training to use public transportation. Also, consider asking if it's possible to work at least part of the workweek at home, so that fewer days are needed at the workplace. An employer that wants you may be your best resource to overcome this barrier.

FUNDING FOR ADAPTIVE AIDS

Job accommodations can be minimal with low cost, but in some cases, changing the work environment to meet an employee's needs can be expensive for smaller employers. Such adjustments that employers can make are designed to help people with low vision or no vision perform their job as well as their sighted coworkers. As visually impaired people have the same working rights as anyone else, employers are expected to make these adjustments in the workplace for their visually impaired employees.

Possible Solutions

If the recommended accommodations are expensive

and beyond the employer's resources, there could be other sources of funding to overcome this barrier. Each state has a state vocational rehabilitation (VR) program. Vocational rehabilitation services are federal-state programs that provide assistance to individuals with disabilities to help prepare for, find, maintain, and advance in employment. (See *Resources*, page 322.) VR also assists businesses in finding, retaining, and advancing employees with disabilities.

The federal part of this program is called RSA (Rehabilitation Services Administration), which was enacted in 1973 as the Rehabilitation Services Act. To access this vital program, simply call the local office in your state and ask to complete an application to determine your eligibility. Upon approval you are assigned your own counselor who may provide funding for accommodations and other services that can lead to employment. The coordination between the employer, vocational rehabilitation services, and yourself is very important to a successful employment result.

NEGATIVE ATTITUDES FROM EMPLOYERS

Another common barrier for people with visual disabilities is that many hiring managers are not fully aware of how much visually impaired people are capable of doing. They may not know about all of the assistive technologies that are available. Employers may be skeptical of how someone who does not drive will get to work. But more than that, some employers may question things like possible lower productivity levels with this new hire and the cost of potential job adaptations.

Possible Solution

The good news is that this barrier can be overcome with education and awareness. An advocate or counselor working on your behalf can coordinate with you and the potential employer during the job-seeking process. Negative attitudes or doubts can change with education and information. It is not always easy, but there are others on your side who can help open doors.

PSYCHOLOGICAL ISSUES

Whether the loss of sight occurs over time or happens quickly, it is not an easy thing to experience. Obviously, it can have a great impact on the way you live your life. Losing your job because of your eyesight's decline is all-too-common. While you may wish to work, the emotional turmoil you may be experiencing can stop you from moving forward. This may be an important and overlooked factor when it comes to the low number of employed people who are visually impaired. It can be a lot to deal with, but there are answers.

Possible Solutions

Having a support group made up of friends and relatives with whom you can talk will help you feel that you are not alone. Contacting a psychologist to help you deal with your feelings can also be an important step. Calling any of the organizations that are set up to assist people in similar situations should be an important consideration.

Blind rehabilitation programs often provide their own individual and group counseling opportunities. Group counseling is important because those involved can share experiences with others who also have a visual impairment. (See *Resources*, page 300.)

There is no question that this can be a tough situation. However, it's important to understand that you are not alone. There are dedicated people and organizations out there that are there to help. Remember, though, that it is sometimes *you* who has to take the first step.

LOOKING FOR THE RIGHT JOB

Since jobs for people with poor vision can vary greatly, it's important to explore occupations and/or careers that are of actual interest to you. There are more than 300 occupational fields that have people with visual impairment on their staff. Finding something that you like and that you feel is rewarding is just as important in your job search as if you were a sighted person. Here are some jobs and careers that you may consider:

■ **Education.** Blind people can work in both traditional school settings and schools for the blind and visually impaired. There are several roles they can fill, both in and out of the classroom. Besides working in a school, they can consider working in a museum or library. Some positions to consider:

- Historian

- Museum educator

- School counselor

- Teacher

- Therapist (speech, physical or occupational therapy)

■ **Business and finance.** Working in this sector would probably mean that you would need some adaptive technology, like a computer with synthesized audio/speech or simple lighting adjustments. There are several career paths to consider with these accommodations. Depending on the role, you may need a bachelor's degree, master's degree, or other types of certifications.

■ **Technology.** Because of all the advances in technology, it's now much easier for visually impaired people to break into the tech sector. This includes working in jobs like coding, engineering, or software development.

■ **Healthcare.** Similar to careers in finance, jobs in healthcare can be performed with little or no vision with the right accommodations and adaptations in the workplace. What's interesting about working in healthcare is that there are several paths to choose from, including mental health, holistic care, or working in a traditional setting.

■ **Answering calls/Making phone calls.** For many companies, the need to have qualified people to provide help over the phone or by computer is important. The same thing is true for people making "blind" sales calls or performing surveys over the phone. With the appropriate training and assistive technological aids, these jobs can be perfect for people who are visually impaired. And in many cases, these jobs can be performed at home.

CONCLUSION

Today, there are many more job and career opportunities for persons who are blind or have low vision than ever before. Assistive technology products and services are readily available to consumers allowing them to educate themselves and secure employment and careers that are fulfilling. Laws such as the American with Disabilities Act in 1990 and the Rehabilitation Services Act of 1973 provide a framework for employers to hire persons with disabilities.

Yes, there have been barriers to employment and some of those barriers are still with us today. The good news, though, is that these barriers continue to fall as most employers see that hiring persons with disabilities is good for business in terms of productivity and job retention.

PART 2

PRODUCTS AND THEIR FEATURES

Today's technology revolution is progressing rapidly in all areas of our lives. Thankfully, this is especially true for low vision and blindness. In Part 2, you will find information on many of the new devices that are already available along with many of the features they may provide. This covers the areas of magnification options, software reading programs, assistive home products, and medical devices.

Reading about what products are available is a good place to start—however, it will be up to you to learn more about the products you may be interested in purchasing. And when you do, make sure that you ask questions, comparison-shop, and check on a product's reviews.

13

Magnification Options

Magnifying lens implements have been used in one form or another by people with poor vision for thousands of years. Today, however, there are a number of new devices that can easily help increase the size of copy for reading or turn written words into spoken language. These range from simple low-tech magnifiers to devices that scan text and read it aloud to the user. This chapter will discuss many of these options.

PORTABLE ELECTRONIC MAGNIFIERS

SMARTPHONES

Smartphones have magnification and zoom features built into both the Android and iPhone operating systems and can be found in the Settings menu under Accessibility. The Accessibility section has programs for persons who are blind (screen reader software) and persons with low vision (magnifier and zoom).

With this built-in software, display and font sizes can also be enlarged, often up to fifteen times (referred to as 15X). The built-in smartphone magnifier function allows for you to zoom in and out of an area with a gesture, using two or three fingers that touch the screen. By simply pinching these fingers together and apart, you can control the size of the magnified area.

In addition to what is already included in your smartphone for magnifying, there are third-party apps that can be downloaded and used to magnify what is displayed by the camera or is displayed on the screen. When viewing print or any physical object, you may also use the flashlight feature for additional lighting as needed. The smartphone magnification and zoom features are similar to the smaller portable electronic magnifiers discussed later in this chapter. The accessibility features are easy to learn how to use. YouTube instructional videos are available for users, if needed.

HANDHELD MAGNIFIERS

This type of low-tech, battery-powered magnifying glass comes in various shapes and sizes. Handheld LED-lighted pocket magnifiers are very popular for many users—and for good reasons. Portable magnifiers are generally small and easy to carry in a pocket or purse. The LED lighting is bright and focuses the light directly on the item or material the user wants to view. Finally, the LED light can be turned off if it's too bright or adjusted to be less bright.

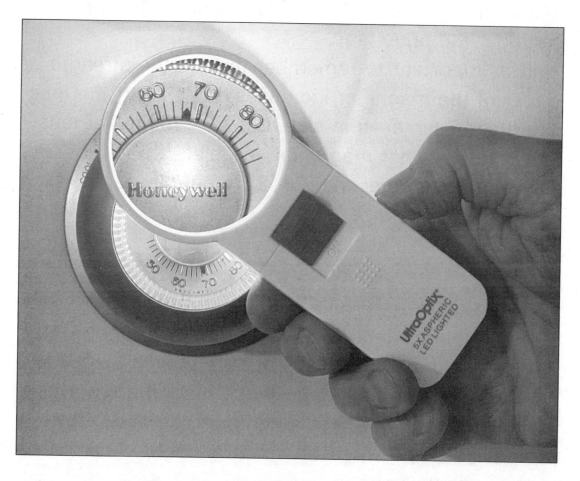

Handheld battery-powered illuminated handheld magnifiers are available in many different strengths. They are small enough to carry in your pocket or purse.

Some instructions can be helpful since the user is working with three items to get the focus set. The user is working with the material or item being viewed, the magnifier lens itself, and finally, the eye of the user.

The user must hold and position the handheld magnifier in order to focus in on what is being viewed. These magnifiers can be used on printed information plus many other items such as wall thermostats, appliance settings, and price tags.

It is important to remember that as the strength or power of the magnifier increases, the size of the magnifier lens decreases in size. So, a 3X magnifier lens—that is, a lens that magnifies an object three times its size—is much larger than an 8X magnifier lens, which is eight times its size.

STAND MAGNIFIERS

Stand magnifier lenses have the same properties as the handheld magnifier lens but are placed on a stand with LED lighting included. These magnifiers are generally larger than pocket magnifiers, so they are less portable, but they are still small enough to carry in a purse or backpack.

When using a stand magnifier, the user places the magnifier directly on the paper, and the focus is automatically set. The LED light has a switch on the stand magnifier, allowing the user to turn the light on or off as needed. These magnifiers are generally used to read printed information but can be placed on flat objects such as currency, coins, or other flat material.

GLOBE MAGNIFIERS

Globe magnifiers, which look much like a paperweight, are also useful. The user simply lays a globe magnifier on the reading material and the magnifier is automatically in focus. These too have different levels of magnification power. These magnifiers do not have LED-lighting options. These are used on printed information.

PORTABLE ELECTRONIC MAGNIFIERS

Portable electronic magnifiers have become very popular since they were introduced in the early 2000s. There are many choices for users. It is best to try out different screen sizes and functions to determine what works best for the user.

Portable electronic magnification devices utilize high-definition cameras, built-in LED lighting, different screen sizes, and in many cases, a reading stand along with voice output/audio options. Built-in rechargeable batteries are designed to provide hours of use before they need to be recharged. By combining enlargement with audio, many users benefit from this dual form of reading.

These devices are available in several different screen sizes. Most units have 4-inch to 10-inch screen sizes. The most common screen sizes are 5-inch and 7-inch. These two sizes usually provide enough magnification while allowing the devices to be easily carried to different locations.

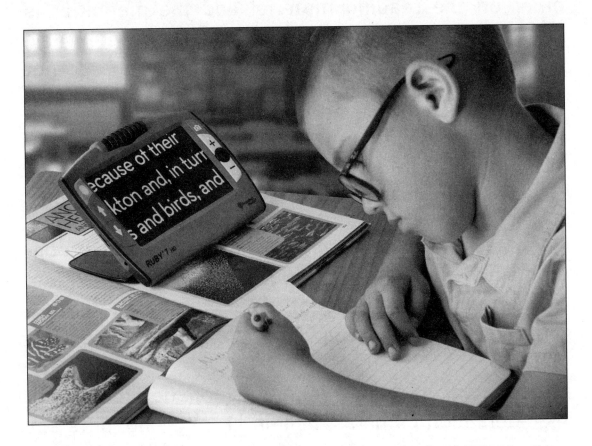

Young student using a portable battery-powered 7-inch electronic magnifier. These devices can easily travel from class to class and then home.

Some manufacturers include optical character recognition—that is, the ability to take a picture of the text and have the text read aloud to the user. These devices have become very popular due to the size, weight, and the ability to easily carry them wherever the user goes. Carrying cases are included, and most devices can operate for several hours once the unit's battery is fully charged. While most portable electronic magnifiers are not designed to write notes easily under the camera, a few come with a writing stand that helps with signatures.

Additional Features

Other common features to be aware of may include the ability to:

- Zoom in and out to change the size of text.

- Change modes, so the foreground and background of the reading material can be changed.

- "Freeze" what is being viewed.

- Tilt the screen for easier viewing.

- Increase and decrease brightness.

- Speak in different languages.

- Alter the rate of speech and volume.

Before purchasing a portable electronic magnifier, make sure to select a device that has the features most important to your needs.

DESKTOP AND TRANSPORTABLE VIDEO MAGNIFIERS

There are two types of video magnifying devices. One is stationary and the other can be moved from place to place. Each can record the item being viewed and enlarged.

DESKTOP VIDEO MAGNIFIERS

Desktop video magnifiers are devices that are produced by various manufacturers in different sizes and configurations. These machines usually have four common features. First, they come with a high definition camera combined with a larger monitor, and built-in lighting. Second, the video magnifier, often referred to as a closed-circuit television (CCTV) system, uses a stand-mounted or handheld video camera to project a magnified image onto a built-in video display, a television screen, or a computer monitor. Third, the cameras come with zoom lenses that provide variable sized magnification. And last, their controls are positioned on the desktop unit for easy access.

In most of these systems, magnification level and focus are set after choosing a comfortable and functional working distance between the camera and the material to be viewed. Many machines are produced with 24-inch monitors and are placed upon a desk or table and are not often moved due to their size and weight. Smaller monitor sizes are also available.

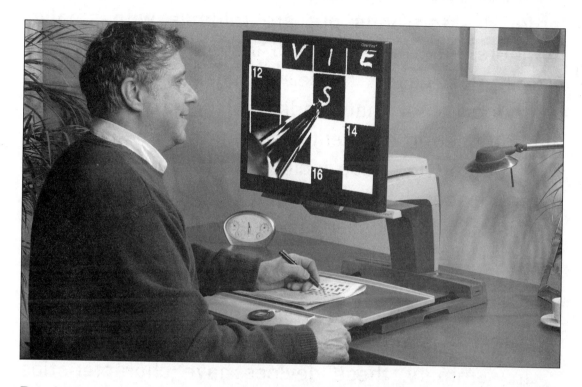

Desktop low-vision machines can be used to read text, labels on cans, and complete puzzles. In addition, users can easily write notes, checks, and complete crossword puzzles.

CCTVs that have cameras are mounted in a fixed position that requires the reading material to be placed under the camera. However, the platform that the material is placed on is movable. It can move from the top of the page to the bottom and side to side. These platforms are usually referred to as an X-Y table. Stand-mounted cameras are particularly effective for handwriting because a hand can fit under the camera.

TRANSPORTABLE VIDEO MAGNIFIERS

Transportable video magnifiers look much like the larger desktop units but are foldable with smaller monitors, anywhere from 15 inches to 17 inches in size in most cases. These machines are designed to be much lighter than traditional desktop units and may be used in different locations by transporting it with the carrying case included with purchase. Often these devices have rechargeable batteries included and, in many cases, can view items in the distance by pointing the camera toward what the user wants to view. Self-viewing is often included allowing the user to point the camera at their face which can help in applying makeup.

In summary, these devices have characteristics similar to full-sized desktop low-vision machines, but they are:

■ Much lighter in weight.

■ Easily transportable with a carrying case.

■ Equipped with rechargeable batteries.

■ Able to provide three different viewing modes (distance viewing, self-viewing, and the viewing of written material).

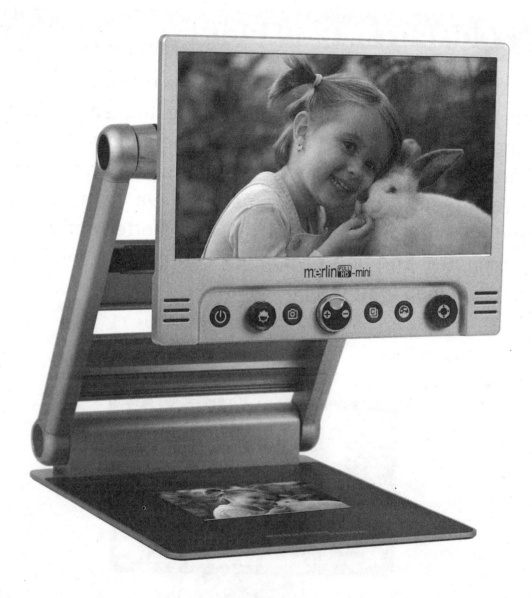

Using a lightweight portable low-vision machine in the self-viewing mode. In this mode, users can point the camera toward themselves and apply makeup.

COMPUTER ENLARGING/ACCESS

For those with low vision, the ability to use a computer can be challenging—from controlling the settings to being able to see what appears on the screen. To help overcome these common problems, magnification software and hands-free glasses have been developed. These products allow the user better access to a computer. The use of speech can also be included and combined with magnification.

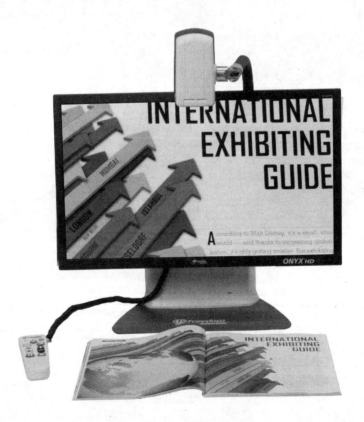

A desktop low-vision machine that has a camera with more flexibility. The camera can view objects in the distance, as well as pages of text.

MAGNIFICATION SOFTWARE

A common way for low-vision computer users to enlarge the text and images displayed on the monitor/display is to use either built-in or third-party zoom software, combined with a larger monitor.

Built-in Magnification Software

The computer operating systems have zoom software that is already built into the Settings menu that enlarges text and images. The zoom feature works by magnifying the items on the screen, and the magnification can be adjusted in size to fit the user's needs. The features of zoom software can be activated and altered using voice recognition, rather than your keyboard and mouse pointing device if you prefer.

The zoom magnification software that is free and part of the operating system of your computer is basic but should meet the needs of many users. It has many features found in zoom software purchased from third-party vendors.

Third-Party Software

In addition to what is already built into computers, third-party software products such as *ZoomText*, Fusion, and SuperNova magnifier software may be purchased and used as well. Both software products have many advanced features that enhance what is viewed.

The magnification software programs that can be purchased have many advanced low-vision features. These include cursor enhancement, mouse enhancements, preferred format with which to display the enlarged text, different foreground and background colors, screen-reading, and many more. The user decides what features are most useful for their needs. The user can then select those features to always be available as part of the default start-up each time the computer is turned on.

Instruction can be provided to assist users in selecting features that work well for themselves. Demo versions can be used prior to buying these products.

VIRTUAL REALITY HEADSETS (VR HEADSETS)

You may be aware of headsets that can be worn over one's eyes in order to play "virtual reality" games, where a player can see a world that does not exist. The same devices may also be used to enhance low vision. Companies that offer these VR devices to low-vision users typically add specialized software to the device that enhance the magnification and speech features. With its built-in camera to collect images from the outside world, it can then send them to the display area within the headset. The software that these VR headsets use can zoom in, zoom out, and even alter the acquired pictures, which allows these headsets to serve as low-vision aids.

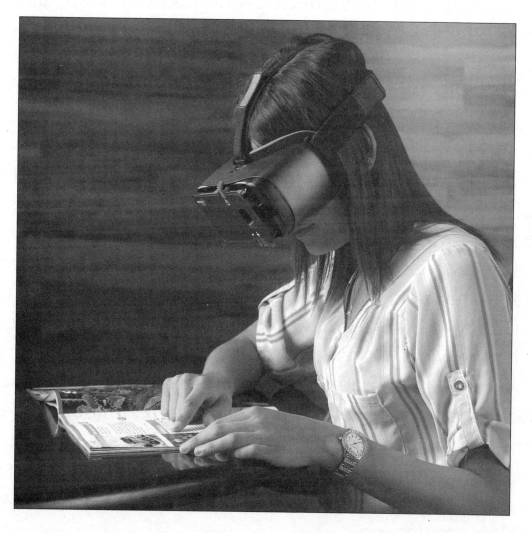

The above photo illustrates the use of a VR headset—a head-worn electronic device—that enlarges the text and images in addition to providing Optical Character Recognition (OCR) functions, which will read the text aloud to the user.

Many VR headsets can be controlled by three methods: One, their eye-tracking programs allow you to control what you are looking at through your *own* eye movements. Two, they can also follow the movement of your hands, which acts like the handheld mouse still used with most desktop computers. And lastly, they can be controlled through voice commands.

While these low-vision aids are advised for use especially for people with serious vision problems such as age-related macular degeneration (AMD) and diabetic macular oedoma (DMO), they may not work properly for some eye disorders. These aids, equipped with advanced virtual reality components, help those people with low peripheral vision or central vision to carry out daily activities more easily by offering an additional field of view. This provides the means with which to magnify fonts, making it far easier for those with low vision to read comfortably.

Many options are included, such as optical character recognition (OCR), which will read text aloud. Other options include placing apps on the screen, zooming, changing modes, and being able to adjust Brightness levels. Training may be needed for electronic low-vision eyeglasses.

Wearing these headsets may not be for everyone. The images that appear in these headsets can be somewhat confusing—even disorienting—to some users. Most manufacturers do not recommend that users walk anywhere while wearing these devices. Furthermore, and because many of these headsets weigh over one pound, it may take some time to get accustomed to using a device like this.

For some, it can cause eyestrain after being worn for only a few hours, and some devices need to be recharged frequently—usually after three to four hours' use. The retail prices for these headsets range from several hundred dollars to several thousands of dollars. So, before you consider purchasing a VR headset, make sure you test it out in your home and work environment—and ask how long you may have to return it, in case it doesn't work for you.

BIOPTIC LENSES

Bioptic lenses, also called bioptic telescopic lenses, or more informally known as "bioptics," are a pair of specialized lenses that are used to improve vision. They consist of two lenses with one or two small telescopes that are fixed to an existing set of eyeglasses. The telescope is fixed a little above your usual line of sight.

One of the main benefits of these lenses is that they help you see things that are much farther away. For example, if your normal vision allows you to see only up to ten feet away, a bioptic lens that can increase your vision times four (4X power) will help you see clearly up to distances of about forty feet.

Bioptic lenses are commonly used to help drivers with low vision see road signs and traffic lights positioned at a distance that they would usually not be able to see. They are like miniature binoculars that can be used either for one or both of your eyes. Bioptic lenses must be prescribed by a licensed optometrist or ophthalmologist.

If you are planning to use bioptics to help you drive, you will likely need extensive training to make the best use of these lenses. You should also be aware of the regulations in your state to know if you can qualify to drive with bioptic lenses based on your current vision. It's best to check with your local licensing agency or department to know where you stand. (See Chapter 7, *Traveling Outside Your Home*, page 101 and *Resources*, page 329 for more information.)

ENHANCEMENTS TO MAGNIFICATION

Along with magnifiers, there are other things you can use to help improve your ability to work on any of these monitor-based devices. This includes the following:

■ **Task lighting** is lighting that focuses the light directly on what the user wishes to view. Task lighting most often is a desk or stand lamp. The type of light coming from the bulb can project a warm atmosphere by providing a red, orange, or yellow hue. Alternatively, the lamp can emanate a light that provides a cool atmosphere by giving off a bluish or white glow. This is, of course, an individualized choice. Proper lighting will affect your viewing comfort and reduce eye fatigue.

Overhead lighting that illuminates the entire room or specific work area can often create a glare on the monitor/display. Consider repositioning the monitor to a location that has no glare on the screen.

■ **The size of the monitor** is also a factor to consider when you access information on your computer. Generally, larger monitors are most helpful for enlargement. A larger monitor and improved lighting may allow a user to see text well with the benefit of using lower levels of magnification than previously required.

■ **Audio voice output** can enhance the text being viewed by the low-vision user. The low-vision software mentioned previously offers speech/voice designed to combine with magnification. Combining enlargement and voice/audio output are an excellent way to continue using and accessing a computer for low-vision users.

■ **Computer keyboards** can be modified by applying large-print letters and numbers on the keys. The foreground and background colors of these letters can be white on black, black on white, yellow on black, and other combinations. In addition, tactile material such as small pieces of velcro or raised dots may be applied to the keyboard's keys, providing a way for the user to keep their hands oriented to the home row on their keyboard.

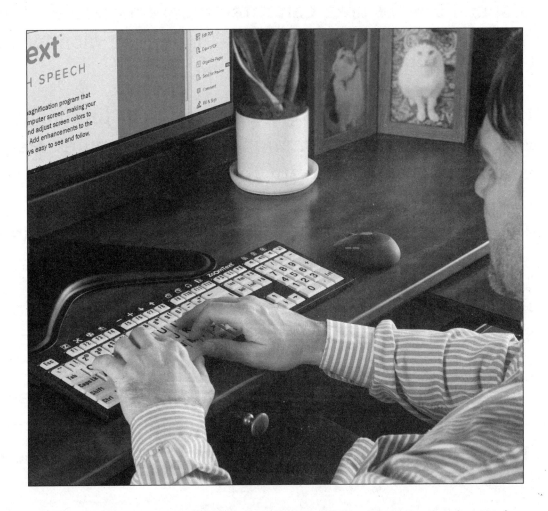

Example of a keyboard with larger, bolder letters and numbers. Users may also include tactual marks on certain keys to help with typing accuracy.

In addition, large-letter keyboards are also available to replace the standard keyboard. While it takes a little practice to get used to the wider finger placement on the larger keyboard, it can be helpful.

■ **Computer training** may be necessary to use computer equipment and software programs. Since many machines require different methods to operate, it is a good idea to select a program that works best for you. Training may consist of audio training modules or professional one-on-one training by a computer access expert. An accommodation expert can evaluate the user's needs and make recommendations.

CONCLUSION

For those with low vision, the ability to magnify an image can make all the difference in the world. While it is certainly no cure, it enables people with poor sight to once again see the things that are important to them—from reading a newspaper to turning on a dishwasher to seeing pictures of their family. This chapter will hopefully let you find the software or device that is best for your own needs.

14

Software Reading Programs

Today, computers come in many shapes and sizes. They can be a traditional larger desktop computer, a smaller portable laptop computer, an even smaller tablet, and finally, a smartphone. They allow us to access the internet, send emails, sign electronic documents, read our local or national newspapers, manage our money, and so much more. These devices can also be of great assistance to those who are visually impaired. By knowing what settings are available within each device, they can easily be turned on to meet the needs of their visually challenged users.

The question then is: What settings come with what devices? To answer that question, we have to know what program a computer device runs on. Most of these devices run on one of three different operating systems—they are Apple-, Windows-, or Android-based devices. And within each of these systems, there are built-in settings specifically designed to help people with visual loss. In this chapter, we will discuss what these settings are for each of these operating systems as well as those that can be added to your device.

APPLE PRODUCTS

Apple hardware is accessible for most people with disabilities straight out of the box and does not require the purchase or installation of extra adaptive software. Apple uses their own software to operate all of their products. You can buy the latest Apple device and have it set up within minutes. Of course, if you need help, just ask the person selling the device to help you turn on any of these settings. All Apple devices (Mac computers, iPads, and iPhones, among others) have the following built-in programs for individuals with disabilities:

■ **VoiceOver.**

VoiceOver is a text-to-speech and screen-reader feature that allows the Apple device to read the text on the screen once the setting is turned on. It can also provide audible descriptions of what's on the screen, such as which app your finger is on, who may be calling you, and the level on your smartphone's battery. In addition, it can adjust the rate of speech and the pitch of the voice.

Available on: iPhone, iPad, Mac, Apple Watch, Apple TV+, and HomePod.

■ Zoom.

Zoom is a screen magnification feature built into Apple products. It should not be confused with the face-to-face internet virtual meeting service also called Zoom. It can customize the size of your text on the screen. It can also increase whatever image is on your screen up to 15 times its original size. Additional features include bolding text and inverting colors, such as white text on a black background.
Available on: iPhone, iPad, Mac, Apple Watch, and Apple TV.

■ Live Speech.

Another Apple feature that may help is called Live Speech. You type in what you want to say, and your device will speak it out loud, so you hear what you type. You are able to save commonly used phrases to respond with during daily interactions or while having lively conversations with friends and loved ones. You can also adjust the voice you want to use, including your own.
Available on: iPhone, iPad, Mac, Apple Watch, and Apple TV.

■ Magnifier.

The magnifier setting works like a digital magnifying glass. It uses the camera on your iPhone or iPad to increase the size of any physical object at which you point it, like a menu or sign, so you can see all the details clearly on your screen. Use the flash to light the object, adjust filters to help you differentiate colors, or freeze a specific frame to get a static close-up. So the magnifier feature provides a tool to read information NOT on your screen.

Available on: iPhone, iPad.

■ Dictation.

This setting lets you type by speaking—and it works in more than 60 languages. To turn your speech into text, just tap the microphone button on the onscreen keyboard in any text field or activate Dictation through System Settings on your Mac.

Available on: iPhone, iPad, Mac, Apple Watch, Apple TV.

In summary, Apple products have adaptive software built into the products they manufacture. The adaptive software features are found within the computer settings and then activated by choosing to use any feature you may need. There is no extra cost to you to access these features and use them.

OTHER SOFTWARE PROGRAMS

Besides the Apple products and the software that Apple provides, there are other very common hardware and software programs that you might want to use. Most people have heard of the popular product called Windows, which also has software built in for blind and low-vision users. This includes magnification, screen reading, and features for users who have difficulty using a standard keyboard and/or mouse. Windows is used on many different desktop and portable computers.

The most common software system for portable and mobile smartphones and tablets is called Android, which is a Google-based product. Phones and tablets that use Android also have settings to assist blind and low-vision users.

WINDOWS

A Windows computer will be identified as such in the specifications listed for the computer. If the computer is identified as an Apple Mac computer, then it will not be a Windows computer. A buyer needs to locate and read the specifications for any computer they may want to purchase. Windows 11 software also has a full range of built-in accessibility features, much like

Apple computers and devices. These too are designed to empower every user. These functions are turned on or off in the Settings menu of the computer that you use. It is possible you may need assistance to learn how to independently use the Menu system to access these features. Let's explore some of these features:

■ **Narrator.**

This is Windows' built-in screen reader. It simplifies navigation, describes images using a natural human-sounding voice, and works seamlessly with supported braille devices. You can use Narrator to read aloud text in a document or email, in an application, on the web, or on the screen. Turn on the functionality when inside a webpage, document, or file.

■ **Color control.**

Windows 11 offers dark and contrast themes that allow you to adjust for light and color sensitivity. You can reduce screen brightness and increase contrast without compromising quality.

■ **Magnifier.**

For low-vision users, you may tailor your screen experience by adjusting cursor size, text size, color, and more. Additionally, you can zoom in on words and images using the magnifier tool.

■ Voice typing.

Convert your speech to text using AI. Windows 11's voice-typing feature even takes care of punctuation.

■ Immersive Reader.

The Immersive Reader allows you to listen to the text read aloud or to adjust how the text looks by changing the space, color, and more on the screen. It enhances online reading fluency, comprehension, and focus.

Whether you are visually impaired, hard of hearing, or have other accessibility needs, Windows 11 offers a comfortable and inclusive experience. There is no extra cost for these features. They are built into the system, much like the Apple accessibility programs.

ANDROID PHONES AND TABLETS

Android is a mobile operating system developed by Google to be primarily used for touchscreen devices, cell phones, and tablets. Its design lets users manipulate the mobile devices using simple finger movements such as pinching, swiping, and tapping. The software programs for Android devices are usually referred to as "apps" (short for applications). Below are some apps that may be used. New apps are constantly being developed and made available, so try to keep up-to-date.

■ TalkBack.

TalkBack is one of many accessibility features on Android intended for users who are blind, have low vision, or otherwise have difficulty seeing the contents on a phone's screen. TalkBack provides verbal feedback that explains what's on the screen, along with vibrations when interacting with it. It makes it possible to use the device without looking at it.

When TalkBack is activated, you can highlight different onscreen elements, and it will read text aloud to you or otherwise describe those elements. Also, it changes the way you navigate your phone. To activate elements, you have to tap twice, and you can also unlock access to a variety of features by using gestures and swipes with multiple fingers at a time. Some training is needed to learn the commands.

■ ShinePlus app.

An add-on app for Android is ShinePlus App. It has these features:

- **Screen reading.** ShinePlus reads out the content on the screen, making it accessible to users who cannot rely on visual cues.

- **Magnification.** It also provides magnification capabilities, allowing users to enlarge text and other elements for better visibility.

- **Language support.** ShinePlus supports multiple languages.

- **Available free.** You can download the ShinePlus app for free from the Google Play Store.

■ Be My Eyes.

Be My Eyes is a mobile app with one main goal: To make the world more accessible for blind and low-vision people. The app connects blind and low-vision individuals with sighted volunteers from all over the world through a live video call. This app works on both Android and Apple iOS products.

Launched in January 2015, Be My Eyes has over 7 million volunteers signed up to assist blind and low-vision users. Be My Eyes is more than a reading app. Its users can request assistance in over 180 languages, making the app the biggest online community for blind and low-vision people as well as one of the largest micro-volunteering platforms in the world.

Each day, volunteers sign onto the Be My Eyes app to lend their sight to blind and low-vision individuals to tackle challenges and solve problems together. Volunteers decide the days and hours they make themselves available to assist a low-vision user.

Here is one example of assistance that could be used with the Be My Eyes app: The low-vision user calls a volunteer with their smartphone and requests to have a printed recipe sitting on their kitchen counter read aloud by the sighted volunteer to the low-vision user. The low-vision user then points their smartphone camera toward the printed recipe so that the sighted volunteer can see it and be able to read it aloud.

■ Seeing AI app.

This app is designed for the blind and low-vision community. It harnesses the power of Artificial Intelligence (AI) to assist users in the navigation of their day. The Seeing AI app is available in both Android and Apple iOS platforms, making it accessible to a wide range of users. Here are the key features of Seeing AI:

- **Object recognition.** Point your phone's camera at objects, and the app will audibly describe them to you. It can recognize and narrate various items, including people, text, currency, color, and general objects.

- **Text reading.** Seeing AI can instantly read short snippets of text as soon as they appear in front of the camera. Additionally, it provides audio guidance to capture full documents, making it useful for reading printed pages.

- **Barcode scanning.** The app can scan barcodes and provide guided audio cues to identify products. This feature is handy for shopping or identifying items.

• **Facial recognition.** Recognize and locate faces of people you are with, along with facial characteristics, approximate age, and even perceptible emotional responses.

• **Scene description.** Using the power of AI, Seeing AI describes scenes around you. It turns the visual world into an audible experience, providing context and information.

• **Currency identification.** The app can identify currency bills whenever you choose to pay with cash.

THIRD-PARTY PRODUCTS FOR COMPUTERS

There are third-party products that are available for Windows computer users if the Windows built-in accessibility programs are not as effective as you want them to be. Here are some examples of what can be added and/or purchased for your Windows desktop or laptop computer.

■ JAWS.

A screen reader for blind users to consider is JAWS (Job Access With Speech). JAWS is a powerful full-featured product that is constantly being revised to work with the latest computer application programs.

It is designed especially for employment opportunities and students.

Available from: Freedom Scientific website.

■ **Fusion.**

Fusion software contains JAWS, but also adds on ZoomText low-vision software so that you have both JAWS screen reader combined with ZoomText low-vision software.

Available from: Freedom Scientific website.

■ **ZoomText Magnifier/Reader.**

ZoomText Magnifier/Reader is a fully integrated magnification and reading program tailored for low-vision users. Magnifier/Reader enlarges and enhances everything on your computer screen, echoes your typing and essential program activity, and automatically reads documents, webpages, and email.

Available from: Freedom Scientific website.

■ **OpenBook.**

OpenBook software is a scanning and reading system that instantly converts printed materials to speech or large-print output on your computer that runs Windows. OpenBook gives you access to what you need to read, whether it's a book, classroom assignment, bill, or PDF document. All you need is a scanner connected to your Windows computer.

Available from: Freedom Scientific website.

CONCLUSION

Today, your desktop computer, laptop computer, tablet, or smartphone have the ability to read text aloud to you using a built-in software screen reader as well as being able to magnify the text. Using these adaptive features will allow you to continue interacting with the world through emails and internet websites. It is important to know that the built-in apps that come with your device, along with the add-on apps from the App store, are continually being improved and revised to work better and more efficiently.

In many cases, online tutorials are available for you to learn more about all of these features and apps so that you can take full advantage of what each program can do for you. Networking with other users should also help you to remain current with new products being developed, as well as improved versions of adaptive software.

15

Connecting to Your Assistive Products

Many of the voice-activated devices available in your home today—such as the ones described in the next chapter—require a common controlling program based on Wi-Fi to operate. There are currently four companies that provide such a service—they are Amazon, Apple, Google, and Samsung. Each of these companies requires an app to be installed on a smartphone and/or computer device. They can also be tied into a separate voice-activated control unit called a *hub*.

In some cases, the assistive devices that receive the commands must be a product associated with or manufactured by one of these companies. For some products, the manufacturer has enabled their devices to work with more than one of these companies' programs—or they can work independently.

While the apps these companies provide are free, the devices these are tied into cost money—from the purchase and installation of the equipment to a potential monthly charge for a specific service.

Amazon Alexa

As mentioned earlier in this book, Amazon Alexa is a cloud-based voice assistant that can perform a variety of tasks. Using Artificial intelligence (AI), it can answer questions, set reminders, play music, and control smart home devices. It requires the purchase of the Echo, which is its voice-activated control unit. It can then be hooked up to control other Amazon products, as well as other third-party manufactured products.
Website: https://alexa.amazon.com

Apple HomeKit

The Apple Homekit, also called Apple Home, is a virtual assistant software app that can control various Apple-interfaced smart products such as lights, temperature, locks, security cameras, and other automated devices. While the app is free, there is a cost involved in setting up each product interface. Homekit works on iPhone, iPad, HomePod, and the Apple Watch. There is also a HomeKit hub, which acts as a voice-activated digital assistant.
Website: https://apple.com/shop/accessories/all/homekit

Google Assistant

The Google Assistant is a free virtual assistant software app that is available on mobile smartphones and can be used on home automation devices. While the app is free, there are costs involved in buying products that interface with Google Assistant. Using Artificial Intelligence (AI), Google Assistant can engage in conversation with its user or allow a user to provide instructions to Google assistive products. It can be used on the Google Home hub, as well as on the Android 5.0 and 6.0 or higher smartphones.
Website: https://assistant.google.com

Google Home

Google Home, also called Google Nest, is both a free app that is available on mobile smartphones and as a voice-activated smart speaker that acts as a digital assistant, much like Amazon's Echo. While the app is free, there are costs involved in buying products that interface with Google Home. It too uses Artificial Intelligence (AI). Google Home can engage in conversation with its user or allow a user to provide instructions to Google assistive products. In addition to working on its voice-activated speaker, it can also work on Android 5.0 and 6.0 or higher smartphones.
Website: https://home.google.com/welcome

Samsung SmartThings

SmartThings is a free app that uses Wi-Fi to connect smart devices built on a Matter protocol. This Matter protocol program allows smart home devices, regardless of the company that makes them, to work with each other through this app. The SmartThings app is available for both iOS and Android. And while SmartThings turns your phone into a control center for all of the smart devices to which it connects, there is also a SmartThings hub that can act as a voice-activated digital assistant.

Website: www.samsung.com/us/smartthings

As it turns out, the technological advances brought forth by these companies have truly changed the way life can be lived by those with low vision and blindness. Of course, these advancements come with periods of frustration—from getting your smart lock to work right to telling your dishwasher to turn on—but once these things work, life can and will be better. As you will learn in the next chapter, the age of smart devices is here, and connecting them to how we live our lives should be the next step.

16

Assistive Home Products

As we discussed earlier in Part 1, there are many assistive devices available to help you live well in your home. These include safety devices, entertainment, lighting, heating, and devices to aid you in your kitchen and laundry room.

The purpose of this chapter is to give you the characteristics of smart devices that may help you in your home. As you choose them, consider these features: audio feedback, voice control, and compatibility with other smart home devices such as Amazon Alexa or Google Assistant. Always keep in mind that whatever smart device you choose, the product and its corresponding app must be "user-friendly" and should meet your needs.

SMART HOME SAFETY SYSTEMS

Smart home safety systems for individuals with low vision incorporate features that enhance accessibility—

and provide peace of mind. Here are some components and systems that can be included in a smart
home safety setup.

FRONT DOOR PROTECTION

If you are alone in your home and you have poor vision,
you will want to have a safe way to identify the person
knocking at your door. There are a number of security
programs to consider. These include the following:

Front Door Recognition Devices

Your front door lock can be hooked up to a smart lock
recognition program.

■ **Voice-activated.** Door locks can be voice-activated
to unlock on command using not only your own voice,
but also others you wish to have access into or out of
your home.

■ **Bio-identification.** The lock sensor can have a fingerprint touchscreen placed above the doorbell to allow
those who have recorded their fingerprint into the program's memory to have the door automatically unlock.
The system can also be based on facial recognition.

■ **Integrating smart locks to smart home safety systems.** The lock's software can be tied into an overall
command program like Amazon Alexa, Google Home,

and Apple HomeKit to allow you to ask the person at the front door who they are. If you know that person, you can tell the device to unlock the front door.

■ **Smartphone link.** You can install a wireless video doorbell to see and record who is at the door. These devices can be linked to a smartphone, so you can communicate with the person without having to open the door. You can also ask who it is, once you get an alert on your smartphone, even if you are not at home. In addition, the video of the person outside can then be sent to a friend or neighbor who can then tell you who that person is through a phone call.

Most, if not all of these voice-activated locks can be integrated into Alexa, Google Home, and Apple Watch. They also come with physical keys and may also use your fingerprint as a key to open and lock your door. Be aware that they are expensive to purchase and install. Make sure you understand how the system works and that you have a service warranty.

OVERALL HOME SAFETY DEVICES

While it is always wise to know who is at your front door, burglars may not use front doors to gain access into a house. With the appropriate security system in place, you can have the peace of mind that comes with knowing you have a reasonable deterrent against a break-in. And just as important is having both smoke and carbon monoxide detectors in place.

Smart Cameras Alarm Systems

Smart cameras can be placed at the front door, around the outside of the home, or inside the home. When they detect any movement within their range of vision, they inform the homeowner that there is some type of movement taking place outside or inside the home. These images can be viewed on monitors inside the home or on smartphones. They can also be recorded for later viewing. When used as an alarm, they can be programmed to call others outside the home—from neighbors and friends to the local police.

Many of these systems can be made voice-controlled, and compatible with other smart home devices such as Amazon Alexa or Google Assistant.

Smart Smoke and Carbon Monoxide Detectors

Smoke detectors can be connected to your smart home system and provide vocal alerts if smoke or gas is detected. They can also be connected to your smartphone, which can be used to silence the alarm through a verbal command.

INTERIOR CONSIDERATIONS

As we will learn, there are a number of factors that we should consider when changing the setup of your home or apartment to deal with low vision. Making these changes is not always easy. In some cases, it can be time-consuming and costly. It can also be frustrating, as you try to deal with workmen while also learning how to use a new device. The end result, however, should hopefully be a better and safer environment. The following tips should provide you with some important points to consider as you move forward.

SMART THERMOSTATS

Smart thermostats designed for individuals with low vision typically feature voice controls, large and tactile buttons, and clear audio feedback to ensure ease of use. Here are some options and features to consider:

■ **Voice control.** Look for thermostats that offer clear voice feedback and can be controlled through voice commands.

■ **Tactile buttons.** Thermostats with raised, well-spaced buttons can help users identify controls by touch.

■ **Remote access.** Some smart thermostats can be controlled via smartphone apps, which may offer accessibility features for low-vision users.

■ **Compatibility.** Ensure the thermostat is compatible with your heating and cooling system.

■ **Wiring.** Ask if the thermostat you select requires a C-wire, for power, or if it can operate on batteries, as this can affect installation and usage. C-wires ensure compatibility for the installation of all smart thermostats.

SMART LIGHTING

Smart indoor lighting can be an important factor for helping people with low vision. It can be used in every room in a house or an apartment including closets. Here are some key points to consider when looking for smart indoor lights suitable for low vision:

■ **LED lights.** They are both efficient and durable, and can provide a bright field of light. LED lights are recommended for task lighting—that is, where focused light is needed.

■ **Adjustable fixtures.** Having an adjustable lamp allows you to direct the light exactly where it's needed, which is crucial for task lighting.

■ **Voice-controlled Off and On switches.** These can be connected to smart home systems and controlled via voice commands, which is particularly helpful for those who may have difficulty locating light switches.

■ **Adjusting brightness.** Having the ability to lower or raise the brightness of a light can reduce eyestrain, headaches, and potential difficulty when reading.

■ **Color hues.** The color hue of a light can affect visual comfort. Warmer lights (with reddish hues) tend to be easier on the eyes for general room lighting, while cooler lights (with blue hues) are better for detailed tasks.

One type of light does not fit all. Each of us is different in the way we read, watch TV, or work at our desks. Because of that, the position of a lamp or the brightness of a light can make a difference, especially when faced with low vision. It is therefore important to find the right lighting that works best for you.

BEDROOM SMART DEVICES

Your bedroom can be filled with many voice-activated devices. They can all be set up separately or they can all be controlled through a central command device such as Amazon Alexa, Google Home, or Apple Home-Kit. This can include:

■ **Bedroom lights and lamps.** If possible, adjust your lights onto those areas you use most frequently.

■ **Closet lights.** Make sure you have a bright light, especially if you have a walk-in closet.

■ **Television and radio.** If possible, place your television and radio in an area where you have easy access to make any needed adjustments.

■ **Beds.** Make sure you have a clear path to get to your bed. Should a hospital bed be needed in your homes, be aware that there are hospital beds that can be controlled by voice commands.

SMART BATHROOM DEVICES

Smart devices can greatly enhance the safety and convenience of bathroom use for individuals with low vision. Here are some assistive devices and adaptations that can help:

■ **Adjustable lighting.** Lighting that can be dimmed or brightened according to need can help reduce glare and improve visibility.

■ **Touchless smart faucets.** A smart faucet can be turned on and off by the motion of your hand, along with its speed of flow and temperature. Not only does this provide a "hands-free" process, it is also hygienic.

■ **Smart showers.** Voice-activated shower controls can adjust the water temperature from hot to cold.

■ **Safety rails and non-slip strips.** Installing safety rails and using non-slip strips by the toilet and in the shower can prevent accidental falls.

■ **High-contrast accessories.** Using towels, mats, and switch plates in contrasting colors can help those with low vision navigate the bathroom more easily.

■ **Product identification.** Many products stored on bathroom shelves look alike because of their similar packaging. Unfortunately, tubes of creams, packs of pills, and bottles of liquids can be hard to recognize with low vision. Each of these should have a way of being easily identifiable. This can be done by adding large stickers with the names of the products written on them, or using colored rubber bands or adhesive bumps placed on the products.

■ **Smart medical devices.** Many health-based devices that normally provide hard-to-read results can now offer its information in spoken language, from scales and thermometers to glucose level monitors. (See Chapter 17, *Medical Devices*, page 285 for details.)

SMART LIVING DEVICES

Smart devices can turn your living areas into a more convenient and efficient space. Here are some smart devices that you might consider:

■ **Smart hubs**. Devices like the Amazon Echo, Google Home, or Samsung SmartThings Home Hub act as the central control points for other smart devices throughout our home. (See Chapter 15, *Connecting to Your Assistive Products*, page 267 for details.)

■ **Smart televisions.** A smart TV can connect to the internet and allow you to stream content from various services. It can also be used as a large monitor for your computer.

■ **Smart audio.** High-quality wireless speakers can be placed throughout the house. The speaker can be voice-controlled, using your smartphone or central command hub.

■ **Robot vacuum cleaners.** These self-operating vacuums can be programmed to operate on their own, at certain times, be voice-activated, and repower themselves. They can also be scheduled or controlled by smart hubs.

■ **Smart lighting.** A number of lighting systems allow you to control the lighting in your home by voice command. You are able to make changes in your home and remotely. You can also change colors, and set off and on schedules.

KITCHEN DEVICES AND APPLIANCES

Smart kitchen devices can be incredibly helpful for individuals with low vision, making cooking and other kitchen tasks more accessible and safer. Here are some smart kitchen devices and tools designed for low vision:

■ **Talking digital food scale.** This device can announce the weight of ingredients, which is helpful for measuring portions without needing to read a scale.

■ **Talking measuring jug.** This type of jug is able to tell you the amount of liquid inside the container. By pressing a button, it can tell you how much liquid there is in the jug.

■ **Liquid level indicator.** This tool can alert you when a cup or pot is nearly full to prevent overfilling and spills. These devices often come with large, easy-to-use buttons and clear audio feedback. Many of these devices can be connected to smart home systems and controlled by voice commands, making them even more convenient to use.

■ **Touchless smart faucets.** A touchless smart faucet allows for hands-free operation, which is not only convenient but also hygienic.

■ **Smart pressure cookers.** The Instant Pot Pro Plus is an example of a smart pressure cooker that can be controlled via an app, making it easier to manage cooking times and settings.

■ **Smart coffee makers.** Coffee makers like the Keurig K-Supreme Plus Smart can be programmed to know exactly how you like your coffee and can be operated remotely.

■ **Talking microwave.** A microwave that announces the time, power level, and cooking status can be very useful for someone with low vision. It can also be controlled through voice commands given to your smartphone or smart assistant such as Google Home, Amazon Alexa, or Apple's Siri.

■ **Smart ovens.** Using Wi-Fi, smart ovens can control all cooking functions and features through voice commands given to your smartphone or smart assistant such as Google Home, Amazon Alexa, or Apple's Siri. When selecting smart kitchen appliances, always consider compatibility with existing devices.

SMART LAUNDRY APPLIANCES

Smart laundry appliances designed for individuals with low vision often include features that make them easier to operate and that provides feedback in various non-visual ways.

■ **Smart washing machines.** These washing machines allow you to use voice commands to start and stop the machine or to schedule the machine to start later.

It can also tell you when the load is done. You can control it on a smartphone app or incorporate it into a smart assistant such as Google Home, Amazon Alexa, or Apple's Siri.

■ **Smart dryers.** These machines have the same control features as can be found on smart washing machines. When purchasing them, be sure to have them work with the matching Wi-Fi program already in your home.

CONCLUSION

Only a few years ago, many of these devices and appliances did not exist. Those people with low vision and blindness had to struggle to overcome the handicap of not clearly seeing the instructions printed on the controls of these products. Now, technology has allowed these devices to work with just the use of your voice—but this is only the beginning. It is, therefore, important to keep on top of the latest breakthroughs in all low-vision-based products.

To find any of the products mentioned in this chapter, please go to the *Resources* section found in the back of this book. There you will find the names, websites, and phone numbers of companies that manufacture these items. In addition, there is a listing of catalog companies that specialize in offering an even wider variety of low-vision products. Be aware, there are also other companies that have not been listed in the *Resources* section. Don't be afraid to shop around. Seek out the best-reviewed products and the best deals.

There are two things to keep in mind when shopping for these devices. The first is cost. In many cases, these products can be expensive—and then there is the cost of installation. Make sure you have a clear idea of what the total cost will be when shopping for any of these items. Many of these products do go on sale. Check a company's website for discounts.

The next is frustration. Once a device has been put into your home, it sometimes does not work the way you had hoped. Make sure to ask for some type of warranty that provides you with some assurance that the product will work properly—or that it can be returned. There is also a learning curve that goes along with the use of any of these products. It may take time to get these things to work correctly. It may take some practice to get it right, but once you do, it should be worth it.

17

Medical Devices

In-home medical devices are intended for users in any environment outside of a professional healthcare facility, such as your home. A user of the medical device can be a patient (care recipient), caregiver, or family member who helps provide assistance in using the device. It can be a permanently installed item or a piece of equipment or software that may be used in many different locations in the house—or even in a car when transported.

It is important to remember that many recommendations on what may be needed and planned for can come from medical doctors, nurses, physical and occupational therapists, and rehabilitation engineers. These professionals often help with the transition from medical facility inpatient settings to the home, so they are aware of medical devices and medical equipment that can help maintain safety and independence.

Here are some examples of common in-home medical devices used by persons with visual impairments.

This is not an exhaustive list but does provide you with resources to begin your search. Some of the products mentioned are listed in the *Resources* section, while additional companies can be looked up on the internet.

MEDICAL ALERT DEVICES

In case of any medical emergency in which you may require immediate assistance, there are several ways to contact help. Dialing 9-1-1 is the universal emergency number that can be called on any cell phone. There are also electric devices that you can wear to call for help as well. Based on your living situation—whether you are living with someone or you live alone—you want a method that better services your needs. Here are a few suggestions to consider.

■ **Landline phone calls.**
When dialing 9-1-1 from a traditional landline, emergency responders can find your exact location even if you don't know your location or you are unable to speak. On cell phones and smartphones, your location is not easily identified. Your phone signal is picked up by a tower, which will not provide the dispatcher with a specific location.

■ Smartphones.

All smartphones, even if they are locked, come with a way to call 9-1-1. The procedure for each smartphone, however, differs greatly based on the phone's manufacturer and model. For example, when using an Apple iPhone you say "Siri, call 9-1-1." You can also press the power button five times, and this will dial 9-1-1 automatically. To get this information for your own smartphone, contact the store you purchased your phone from or you can find it on the internet.

■ Medical alert systems.

There are several companies that produce medical alert systems, such as Bay Alert Medical, MedicalAlert, ADT, Lifeline, GetSafe, and Medical Guardian. They normally include a stationary monitor, an app, and a mobile device you wear or carry with you. Once you press the button on the mobile device, it alerts the monitor and/or app to call their dispatcher who then calls 9-1-1 on your behalf. You can also arrange to have the dispatcher call others such as family, friends, police, or first responders. There is normally a monthly fee for this service. To find the service right for you, go online and compare services and costs. Always inquire about possible discounts.

BLOOD PRESSURE MONITORING

There are two types of blood pressure monitors. One forms a cuff around your upper arm, while the other is worn around your wrist. The American Heart Association recommends the cuff monitor as the most accurate. When following the directions provided by the wristband company, the reading can be reasonably close. Just as important, the wrist device can detect important changes—such as elevations and drops in your blood pressure at any time. There are many such devices to choose from, and here are a few to consider:

■ **Apple Watch.**
Your Apple Series 6 and later watches can monitor your blood pressure, your heart rate, and oxygen saturation level. Keep in mind that the Apple Watch blood pressure sensors will not provide exact numbers the same way that the cuff in a doctor's office does.
Available from: Apple stores, Amazon website, and most smartphone outlets, usually at cheaper prices.

■ **Lumiscope Deluxe Auto-Inflate Blood Pressure Monitor.**
The Lumiscope monitor has a large LCD screen that displays systolic and diastolic pressure readings, pulse rate, and a three-color risk indicator. This is a

cuff system that wraps around your arm, however, it does not talk.

Available from: Amazon website and Maxi-Aid catalog/website.

■ **Talking blood pressure monitor.**

This device also uses a cuff system that provides speedy results spoken in English or Spanish.

Available from: Maxi-Aids catalog/website, LS&S catalog/website, and Amazon website.

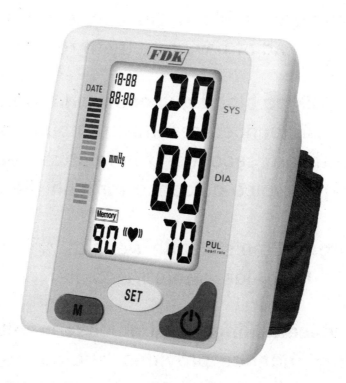

Talking blood pressure meters speak your blood pressure and pulse in a clear male or female voice. Talking blood pressure monitors offer easy operation and have a memory system to retain over 90 measurements.

■ **Reizen wrist talking blood pressure monitor.**
If you prefer a wrist device, the Reizen monitor also offers speech to provide you with the results spoken in English or Spanish.
Available from: Maxi-Aids catalog/website, LS&S catalog/website, and Amazon website.

GLUCOSE MONITORS & DIABETES SUPPLIES

Imagine having your blood glucose levels spoken out loud to you instead of having to try to read a tiny gauge.

■ **Embrace talking blood glucose monitoring system.**
This device announces results in English or Spanish in no more than 6 seconds. It is relatively easy to use by following its voice guidance through the entire test process.
Available from: Omnis Health website, Amazon website, and MaxiAids catalog/website.

■ **Prodigy voice talking blood glucose monitor kit.**
The Prodigy monitor provides audible results and includes control solution, 10 test strips, 10 lancets, and a lancing device.
Available from: Prodigy Diabetes Care website, Amazon website, and MaxiAids catalog/website.

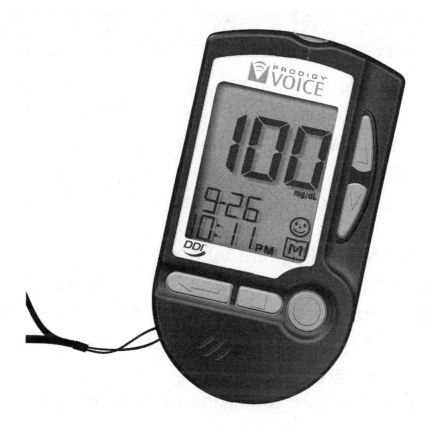

The Talking Glucose Meter is for anyone who is visually impaired. It offers ease of use and provides accuracy with just a small blood sample of blood. Results are announced clearly and records can be stored with the date and time.

■ Prodigy Count-a-dose.

The Prodigy Count-a-dose accurately measures mixed doses of insulin. The unit holds two bottles that are measured into a standard Lo-Dose syringe by turning a wheel that "clicks" for each unit of insulin.

Available from: Independent Living Aids catalog/ website and Amazon website.

MEDICINE AID ORGANIZERS

Never forget your medicine again with medicine aids designed for low-vision and blind persons. Medicine organizers allow you to have your daily medicine already planned out for you. Tools to cut pills and remind you to take your medication are critical.

■ **MEDIPLANNER II.** (Pill Planner/Organizer)
This easy-to-read, extra-large pill planner with 28 extra-large compartments holds 7 days of medication (4 dosages per day). It offers braille and raised letter markings and large bold print.
Available from: from MaxiAids catalog/website.

■ **MedReady 1700 medication pill dispenser.**
(Reminder Product)
Reminder products offer many ways to be reminded of all your important tasks. Whether it's to take medications or to wake up on time, this device provides audio reminders for you and also holds pill medication(s).
Available from: MedReady, Inc. website, Amazon website, and MaxiAids catalog/website.

BLOOD-OXYGEN SATURATION & PULSE RATE

■ Apple Watch.

Your Apple Series 6 and later Apple Watches can monitor your oxygen saturation level, blood pressure, and your heart rate.

Available from: Apple stores, Amazon website, and most smartphone outlets.

■ Talking Pulse Oximeter.

The Talking Pulse Oximeter accurately measures blood-oxygen saturation and pulse rate, and audibly announces the results in English.

Available from: HearMore catalog/website, Amazon website, LS&S catalog/website, and MaxiAids catalog/website.

THERMOMETERS

■ Talking infrared forehead and ear thermometer from Reizen.

Quick one-second temperature readout and twelve memory recalls. It speaks in six different languages: English, German, Italian, Spanish, French, and Russian.

Available from: HearMore website, MaxiAids catalog/website, and Amazon website.

■ **Non-contact infrared talking thermometer.**
This thermometer speaks in English and Spanish. It also has a large backlit digits display in both Fahrenheit and Celsius.
Available from: HearMore website, MaxiAids catalog/ website, and Amazon website.

TALKING AND LOW-VISION SCALES

■ **Talking scales.**
There are now a number of talking scales available; however, most have smaller displays. The Cirbic talking scale has a slightly larger display, but may not be suitable for some with low vision.
Available from: Amazon website and Cirbic website.

■ **Extra-wide 550-pound talking scale.**
This talking scale, with an extra-wide platform, is easy to use and hear. It has a 550-pound capacity and speaks results in pounds or kilograms.
Available from: Independent Living catalog/website.

■ **Extra-large display bath scale.** (for low vision)
Oversized, easy-to-read digital display that measures up to 440 lbs. in 0.2-lb. increments. It has an extra-large, easy-to-read 5.5- x 5-inch display.
Available from: Maxi-Aids catalog/website.

CONCLUSION

The integration of healthcare and safety into the home setting is a growing trend, driven by factors such as rising costs, an aging population, and technological innovations. This shift involves a diverse mix of people, various tasks, and a wide range of devices and technologies. In-home medical devices can help with blood pressure monitoring, diabetic management, safety in the bathroom, weight control, medicine organization, and many more health needs.

Various devices and equipment are available for all of these in-home health needs. The good news is that there are manufacturers of these health devices that provide equipment with low-vision features and are audio/speech-enabled. Remember, when using any home medical device, always follow proper instructions and consult with healthcare professionals on proper use and installation as needed.

Conclusion

While this chapter is called a *Conclusion*, we hope it is just the beginning for those with low vision and blindness. It is not easy losing your sight. It changes your world—from reading a book to looking at a watch. But as it turns out, the revolution in technology has made it possible to overcome many of the barriers that were there only a decade ago. This book was written to open the door to a world that can help you move forward with your life.

In Part 1, we provided an overview of some of the most important areas of your life, such as safety, home living, employment, and finance—things that can assist in carrying out your everyday tasks. In Part 2, we presented the many factors to consider when buying a new device or installing a new technology. And in the *Resources* section, we have listed many of the associations, organizations, manufacturers, and catalog companies dedicated to aiding those with vision impairments. Many of these non-profit groups provide free services and more.

While it is true that a visual impairment can have a profound impact on your life, remember that you are still in control. While we have tried to discuss all the positives that are now available to you, we have also pointed out that there will be times that you will run into problems, likely ones that will frustrate you. You need to be prepared for those moments.

Try to be proactive. Do not be afraid to ask questions. Hopefully, you will get the answers you need. Low vision certainly matters, but the way you live your life matters even more. We hope that this book has been able to answer some of the most important questions you may have had.

Resources

The list of organizations, associations, businesses, and websites you will find under *Resources* are all designed to help people living in the U.S. and Canada with low vision and blindness. The following is a list of the resource categories you will find within this section:

- **General, Financial & Social Services**

- **Healthcare Coverage**

- **Jobs**

- **Scholarships for Careers**

- **Education for Vocations & Independent Living**

- **Guide Dog Providers**

- **Financial Aid for Assistive Products**

- **Manufacturers of Assistive Technology & Adaptive Software**
    - —Assistive Products for the Home
    - —Braille Products
    - —Magnification/Reading Products

—Medical Aids

—Security Devices

—Thermostats

■ **Catalogs & Websites of Low-Vision Products**

GENERAL, FINANCIAL & SOCIAL SERVICES

While this section focuses on national organizations that offer many different services to those with low vision and blindness, there are many regional and local organizations that do the same. Although they may not be listed here, we encourage you to learn more about such groups within your own communities.

ABLE Accounts

(See *Internal Revenue Service (IRS) ABLE Accounts*, page 306.)

Alliance for Equality of Blind Canadians (AEBC)

This national non-profit organization is devoted to raising awareness and supporting equality of its members with low vision, blindness, and blindness with deafness. There are several chapters spread across Canada. If you need assistance in securing your rights, AEBC will find you a disability advocate. They also award scholarships for those with impaired vision who wish to pursue more education. (See also *Alliance for Equality of Blind Scholarship Program*, page 300.)

Website: www.blindcanadians.ca

Phone: 1-800-561-4774

American Council of the Blind (ACB)

The American Council of the Blind is a non-profit organization comprised of 70 state chapters. Guided by its members, ACB advocates for equality of people who are blind and have low vision. It promotes independence of its members through education, resources, and job connections. It awards annual scholarships to outstanding blind post-secondary students. (See also *ACB Job Connection*, page 313 and *ACB Scholarship*, page 316)

Website: www.acb.org
Phone: 1-518-906-1820

American Foundation for the Blind (AFB)

The AFB is a national nonprofit group. Its mission is to increase the independence, security, and equality of opportunity, and quality of life for those with vision loss. It is a strong advocate for the rights of people with low vision and blindness.

It publishes a quarterly online magazine with articles about the intersection of vision loss and assistive technology products. You can find this publication by doing an internet search for "Access World and AFB." This platform connects people with vision loss with others who share similar interests, hobbies, or professions, and offers opportunities for socializing, learning, and mentoring. The AFB also offers scholarships to students. (See also *AFB Scholarship*, page 316.)

Website: www.afb.org
Phone: 1-800-232-5463

American Printing House for the Blind (APH)

The American Printing House for the Blind is a non-profit organization. It provides a wide variety of accessible learning experiences through educational, workplace, and independent living products and services for people who are blind and have low vision. It produces books, magazines, and other publications in braille, large print, or recorded versions as well as educational material. (See also *APH ConnectCenter*, page 302 and *CareerConnect*, page 313.)

Website: www.aph.org
Phone: 1-800-223-1839

APH ConnectCenter

This website is a service provided by the American Printing House for the Blind. It offers three sections: CareerConnect, which provides help for employment; FamilyConnect, which offers support and resources for families and children of the blind and those with low vision; and VisionAwareness, which provides information for people adjusting to blindness or low vision, as well as to family members, and professionals who serve them. (See also *American Printing House for the Blind*, page 301 and *CareerConnect*, page 313.)

Website: https://aphconnectcenter.org
Phone: 1-800-232-5463

BARD (Braille and Audio Reading Download)

A Service of the National Library Service for the Blind and Print Disabled, BARD is a program offered by the National Library Service. It provides a wide selection of audio and braille books along with magazines for school-age children, teens, and adults free of charge. Books are available in English, Spanish, and other world languages. In order to participate in the program, you need to apply for membership on their website and must show proof of vision loss. (See also *National Library Service for the Blind and Print Disabled*, page 308.)

Website: https://nlsbard.loc.gov/nlsbardprod/login/NLS
Phone: 1-888-657-7323

Be My Eyes

This free app on Android smartphones connects visually-impaired people with sighted volunteers or company representatives for visual assistance through a live video call. Sighted volunteers can help with short, simple tasks such as reading a label or checking an expiration date.

Website: www.bemyeyes.com

Blind Veterans Association (BVA)

This group assists eligible blind veterans and their families with VA claims processing and offers assistance programs and services such as help with job securement, peer support, and scholarships. (See also *Veterans Administration*, page 311 and *Blind Veterans Association Scholarship Program*, page 315.)

Website: https://bva.org
Phone: 1-800-669-7079

Braille and Audio Reading Download

(See *BARD*, page 306 and *National Library Service for the Blind and Print Disabled*, page 308.)

Braille Literacy Canada (BLC)

Braille Literacy Canada is a non-profit organization designed to teach braille as the primary medium of literacy for those who are blind or visually impaired. They teach that braille is a writing system and not really a language. BLC's goal is to help all blind persons gain literacy by using braille.

Email: info@blc-lbc.ca
Phone: 1-877-861-4576

Canadian Council of the Blind (CCB)

This non-profit organization works to improve the lives of people who have impaired vision. One of their services is Get Together With Technology (GTT) that provides technology training, by and for people with impaired vision or blindness. Other services include mentoring, socializing, promoting physical activities, maintaining health, and advocacy for those who are blind and visually impaired.

Website: https://ccbnational.net
Phone: 1-877-304-0968

Canadian Federation of the Blind (CFB)

The CFB was organized in 1999 by volunteer blind Canadians to improve and enrich the lives of their fellow blind citizens. The goal is to educate the public as to what it means to be blind. The CFB is a parallel organization to the National Federation of the Blind (NFB) in the United States and has a similar free-cane program called Walking Proud.

Website: www.cfb.ca
Phone: 1-800-619-8789

Canadian National Institute for the Blind (CNIB)

This non-profit organization is dedicated to improving the lives of those Canadians with impaired vision by providing innovative programs and rehabilitation services and resources. This includes hosting special events, such as recreational and social activities, and, gardening discussions. Their guide dog program finds volunteers to raise pups to become guide dogs—and if you are blind, they will also help you find the right guide dog. CNIB also provides youth internships. (See also *CNIB Card*, page 305.)

Website: www.cnib.ca
Phone: 1-800-563-2642

Canadian Organization of the Blind and DeafBlind (COBD)

This charitable organization, headquartered in British Columbia, supports visually impaired persons of all ages to help them achieve independence, dignity, and well-being. It supports summer camps to encourage independence and develop new skills.

Website: www.cobd.ca
Phone: 1-800-264-2623

Care.com

This company's website lists a wide variety of care providers from pet care to housekeeping to senior care. You enter your zip code and answer questions about the types of services you need, how soon, and how many hours. Pictures of possible candidates will appear on the screen and you can then click on them for more information.

Website: www.care.com
Phone: 1-877-227-3115

CNIB Card

If you are legally blind in Canada, you may be eligible for a CNIB Card that is proof of your disability. This card is not obtained from any governmental agency but from the Canadian National Institute for the Blind (CNIB). This card helps you access some government programs and benefits. It also may be used for free or discounted transit, train, air, and bus passes, free or discounted admission to some recreation events, and even access to disability services from banks and other businesses. (See also *Canadian National Institute for the Blind*, page 304.)

Website: www.cnib.ca
Phone: 1-844-887-8572

Family Caregivers Alliance (FCA)

This organization's mission is to improve the lives of family care-givers and the people they care for. They provide state leads to locate public, nonprofit, and private programs and services located closest to the family. These resources include government health and disability programs, legal resources, disease-specific organizations, and more—all designed to help the family cope with the care of a disabled individual. (See also *Payments for Family Caregivers*, page 309.)

Website: www.caregiver.org
Phone: 1-800-445-8106

Internal Revenue Service (IRS) ABLE Accounts

Under the IRS code of the 420(a) section, the IRS allows states to administer Achieving a Better Life Experience Accounts, better known as ABLE Accounts. They are designed to help people with physical disabilities. Just like an IRA account, these accounts allow you to put money into them for investing, and pay no state or federal taxes on the money made in them. Also, there are no taxes or penalties on a withdrawal from the account as long as withdrawals are used to pay qualified disability expenses. You can put up to $15,000.00 a year without having to pay federal taxes, and any money taken out to pay for expenses related to taking care of that disability is also tax-free. (This dollar amount is subject to change, and may increase over time, so check with a financial advisor.)

If you don't believe you qualify for an ABLE account, contact your state's ABLE account program to learn about special deductions you can make or other expenses that you can take relating to your low vision or blindness.

Website: www.irs.gov/government-entities/federal-state-local-governments/able-accounts-tax-benefit-for-people-with-disabilities

Phone: 1-855-004-8300

Lions Club International

Through many of its local groups, the Lions Club provides resources and financial help to people with visual impairments in the U.S. and throughout the world. It also provides funding for organizations that deal with eyecare such as the Lions Eye Bank for Long Island, an independent group providing eye corneas for transplants. In addition, it may provide assistance in home adaptation needs. To learn more about what services are available, you should contact the local Lions Club chapter nearest you. To find the chapter closest to you, go to the website listed below and press the tab titled "Find a club near you."

Website: www.lionsclubs.org

Phone: 1-630-571-5466

Meals on Wheels

Meals on Wheels America is a nationwide volunteer organization located in almost every community in America that delivers daily delicious, nutritious meals to persons over 60 years of age or those who are disabled or those who are housebound and unable to provide nutritious meals for themselves. Although Meals on Wheels is a national organization, each community sets up its own program. To find a local provider, visit the website listed below.

Website: www.mealsonwheelsamerica.org/find-meals

Phone: 1-888-998-6325

Medicare and Medicaid

Medicare is a federal program that offers health insurance for people who are 65 years or older. Medicaid is a federal and state program based upon a limited income. Both programs pay for a wide range of medical services. If you have both Medicare and Medicaid and are visually impaired, you should qualify for better healthcare coverage, lower out-of-pocket costs, and vision and dental care. You may also qualify for long-term care, home healthcare, and prescription drug coverage. (See also *Payments for Family Caregivers*, page 309.)

Medicare/Medicaid Websites: www.medicare.gov/basics/costs/help/medicaid

www.medicaidplanningassistance.org/state-medicaid-resource

Medicare Phone: 1-800-633-4227

National Eye Institute (NEI)

The National Eye Institute (NEI) is part of the U.S. National Institutes of Health, an agency of the U.S. Department of Health and Human Services. Its goal is "to eliminate vision loss and improve quality of life through vision research." The NEI performs and supports vision research, education programs, and clinical trials that protect, prolong, and heal vision.

Website: www.nei.nih.gov

Phone: 1-301-496-5248

National Federation of the Blind (NFB)

This organization of more than 50,000 blind people in the United States is the oldest and largest organization led by blind people in the U.S. NFB's purpose is to promote equal opportunity for the blind and to improve the quality of life of blind people.

The NFB offers various programs and services, such as the NFB-NEWSLINE, a free digital talking newspaper service for the blind and the Blind Driver Challenge, an initiative to develop non-visual interface technology for driving a car in the future. It also offers scholarships to students. The NFB is a parallel organization to the Canadian Federation of the Blind (CFB) in Canada. (See also *National Federation of the Blind Scholarship*, page 318 and *Career Opportunities*, page 313.)

Website: https://nfb.org
Phone: 1-888-882-1829

National Library Service for the Blind and Print Disabled (NLS)

The National Library Service for the Blind and Print Disabled is a free library program of braille and audio materials, such as books and magazines circulated to eligible borrowers in the United States and American citizens living abroad, by sending out postage-free mail and online. (See also *BARD*, page 302.)

Website: www.loc.gov/nls
Phone: 1-888-657-7323

NoisyVision

NoisyVision is a non-profit organization that supports the empowerment of people with low vision and hearing loss and educates the community on topics of accessibility and social inclusion. Through social media, such as Facebook, they provide connected networks for those people with disabilities to share their life stories, experiences, skills, and talents. They also produce videos, publish prose, and promote visual arts and artistic events. In addition, they organize trips to increase the mobility potential of those with visual impairments.

Website: www.noisyvision.org

Payments for Family Caregivers

Several states provide Medicaid programs that allow disabled individuals to recruit, hire, and direct their own home care workers. Some of these programs allow them to hire family members and friends to be their home health aides.

To qualify, the person must have a legally recognized chronic medical condition or physical disability and have trouble with daily living activities or require skilled nursing assistance. In addition, many of these programs are age- and income-based, and require that the individual be a state resident.

Many of these programs have different agency names, so they may be difficult to track down. To learn more, call the agency in your state. Below you will find the name of some states that provide this program, along with the states' service departments and their phone numbers.

If your state name does not appear in the following list, contact your state's department of social services. However, the name for this department may be different in your state. Call your state's Medicare program to get more information as to who to contact.

In addition to these state programs, there are a number of privately owned companies that work with these agencies that can provide individuals needing assistance with the benefits provided under the Medicaid program. (See also *Medicare and Medicaid*, page 307.)

California: The In-Home Supportive Services (IHSS) program
Phone: 1-866-376-7066

Connecticut: Connecticut Dept. of Social Services
Phone: 1-855-626-6632

Florida: Statewide Medicaid Managed Care (SMMC) program
Phone: 1-877-711-3662

Illinois: The Community Care Program (CCP)
Phone: 1-600-252-8966

Indiana: Indiana Dept. of Family and Social Services Administration—Division of Family Resources (DFR)
Phone: 1-800-403-0864

Michigan: The MI Choice Waiver
Phone: 1-734-722-2830

Minnesota: The Consumer Support Grant (CSG) program
Phone: 1-866-267-7655

New Jersey: The Personal Preference Program (PPP)
Phone: 1-609- 631-2481

New York: The Consumer-Directed Personal Assistance Program (CDPAP)
Phone: 1-855-446-3300

Ohio: The PASSPORT program
Phone: 1-614-645-7250

Oregon: The Aged and Disabled Medicaid Waiver
Phone: 503-945-5600

Pennsylvania: The Aging Waiver program
Phone: 1-800-753-8827

Washington: The Medicaid Alternative Care (MAC) program
Phone: 1-800-562-3022

Social Security Disability Insurance (SSDI)

Social Security Disability Insurance (SSDI) benefits depend on your work history and the amount of Social Security taxes, called credits, you have paid in past years. You may also qualify if your parents or spouse have paid Social Security taxes, also called credits. Monthly benefits cover medical care, living expenses, and even rent or a mortgage. The size of monthly payments you would receive depends on the state where you reside. To learn more, contact your local Social Security office, or visit their website, which deals with this subject. (See also *Social Security Supplemental Security Income*, page 311.)

Website for SSDI: www.ssa.gov/disability

Phone: 1-800-772-1213

Social Security Supplemental Security Income (SSI)

A second Social Security program is Supplemental Security Income (SSI), which is based on need. If you have limited or no income and few resources, you may qualify for monthly SSI payments. Under this program you may also qualify for Supplemental Nutrition Assistance Program (SNAP) to pay for food and state benefits like Medicaid to cover medical costs. (See also *Social Security Disability Insurance*, page 311.)

Website for SSI: www.ssa.gov/ssi

Phone: 1-855-532-4556

Supplemental Nutrition Assistance Program (SNAP)

(See *Social Security Supplemental Security Income*, page 311.)

Veterans Administration Visual Impairment Services Team (VIST)

If you are a veteran with low vision or blindness, you may find the Veterans Administration helpful. Contact the Visual Impairment Services Team (VIST) at your nearest VA regional center. They offer rehab and other services to help veterans live an independent life. These include home improvements and structural alterations to make your home more suitable for your vision needs.

In addition, the VA has several Blind Rehabilitation Centers, which are residential inpatient programs that provide comprehensive adjustment to blindness training and serve as a resource to a geographic area usually comprising several states. These centers offer a variety of skill courses designed to help blinded veterans achieve a realistic level of independence. These skill areas include:

- Orientation and mobility
- Visual skills
- Communication skills
- Computer access training
- Activities of daily living
- Social/recreational activities
- Manual skills

On the internet, go to "VA blind and low-vision rehabilitation services" for more information or use the website cited below. (See also *Blind Veterans Association*, page 303 and *Blind Veterans Association Scholarship Program*, page 316.)

Website: www.va.gov/health-care/about-va-health-benefits/vision-care/blind-low-vision-rehab-services

Phone: 1-800-698-2411

Vision Loss Rehabilitation Canada

This health services organization serves people who are blind or partially sighted across the country. Their certified specialists provide training to their low-vision and blind clients to develop or to restore activities of daily living skills, to promote their independence, and to enhance safety and mobility. They work closely with ophthalmologists, optometrists, and other healthcare professionals by providing essential care on a referral basis in homes, workplaces, and communities across Canada.

Website: https://visionlossrehab.ca/en

Phone: 1-844-887-8572

Visions

Visions is a non-profit organization that is designed to assist people of all ages who are blind or visually impaired to lead independent and active lives in their homes and communities. They offer individualized vision rehabilitation training at home or in the community, social services, employment training and job development, and group and community education and activities.

Website: https://visionsvcb.org

Phone: 1-888-245-8333

JOBS

ACB Job Connection

The ACB Job Connection is a service of the American Council of the Blind, which publishes nationwide jobs available under a variety of categories. To learn more, visit their website. (See also *American Council of the Blind*, page 300.)

Website: www.acb.org/jobs

Phone: 1-202-467-5081

Blind Veterans Association (BVA)

(See *Blind Veterans Association*, page 000.)

Career Opportunities

This service from the National Federation of the Blind provides a website for visually challenged people, their families, teachers, counselors, and employers. This site offers job seekers of all ages and employers a variety of resources to help with a job search and hiring process in their community. Visit their website to learn more. See also *National Federation of the Blind*, page 308.)

Website: https://nfb.org/about-us/career-opportunities

Phone: 1-410-659-9314

CareerConnect

CareerConnect is a section within the APH ConnectCenter website that provides information to those in search of employment who have low vision or are blind in search of employment. It is a service

provided by the American Printing House for the Blind. (See *American Printing House for the Blind*, page 301.)
Website: https://aphconnectcenter.org/careerconnect
Phone: 1-800-232-5463

National Industries for the Blind (NIB)

NIB is the nation's largest employment resource for people who are blind and, through its network of associated nonprofit agencies, is the largest employer of people who are blind in the U.S. In addition, they offer career training to provide people with the skills required for manufacturing and professional services careers.
Website: https://nib.org
Phone: 1-703-320-0500

Rehabilitation Services Administration (RSA)

The RSA is a federal agency under the United States Department of Education, Office of Special Education and Rehabilitative Services, and is headquartered within the Department of Education in Washington, D.C. It was established to administer portions of the Rehabilitation Act of 1973. Its mission is to provide leadership and resources to assist state and other agencies in providing vocational rehabilitation (VR) and other services to individuals with disabilities to maximize their employment, independence, and integration into the community and the competitive labor market.

RSA provides formula grants to vocational rehabilitation agencies to administer the VR, supported employment, and the Independent Living Services for Older Individuals Who Are Blind programs (IL-OIB) in all 50 states, the District of Columbia, Puerto Rico, and four U.S. territories. Job training and education are a major focus of this program in each state.
Website: www.rsa.ed.gov/about/states
Phone: 1-800-872-5327

Visions

Visions is a non-profit organization that is designed to assist people of all ages who are blind or visually impaired to lead independent and active lives in their homes and communities. They offer employment training and job placement. (See also *Visions*, page 312.)

Website: https://visionsvcb.org

Phone: 1-888-245-8333

SCHOLARSHIPS FOR EDUCATION & CAREERS

There are many scholarships available for visually impaired students who want to pursue post-secondary education.

25 Great Scholarships for Visually Impaired Students

This website lists the 25 most generous scholarships for visually impaired students. As modern technology continues to make the world an easier place to navigate for individuals with sight-related disabilities, the collegiate campus is also becoming more welcoming to the visually impaired with audio textbooks, touch-based navigation, and easy-access dormitories.

Website: www.top10onlinecolleges.org/scholarships-for/visually-impaired-students

Alliance for Equality of Blind Canadians (AEBC) Scholarship Program

The Alliance for Equality of Blind Canadians (AEBC) scholarship program recognizes outstanding post-secondary Canadian students who are blind, deaf-blind, or partially sighted. (See also *Alliance for Equality of Blind Canadians*, page 300.)

Website: www.royalroads.ca/aebc/allyant-scholarship

Phone: 1-800-788-8028

American Council of the Blind Scholarship Program

The American Council of the Blind offers scholarships that cover tuition fees, room and board, and other additional costs associated with assistive technology for undergraduate, graduate, and technical schools. (See also *American Council of the Blind*, page 300.)

Website: www.acb.org/scholarships

Phone: 1-800-866-3242

Association for Education and Rehabilitation of the Blind and Visually Impaired

This group is made up of professionals who service the blind and visually impaired. The association offers scholarships for the legally blind who are preparing for a career in educating and rehabilitation of blind children and adults.

Website: www.aerbvi.org/resources/aer-scholarships

Phone: 1-703-671-4500

American Foundation for the Blind (AFB) Scholarships

The AFB, in partnership with the American Council of the Blind (ACB), awards students with scholarships to help with post-secondary education financial needs such as tuition, fees, room and board, and other additional costs associated with adaptive technology. Designed for those students attending a technical college or university as an entering freshman, undergraduate, or graduate student. (See also *American Foundation for the Blind*, page 301.)

Website: www.afb.org/about-afb/awards/scholarships

Phone: 1-800-232-5463

Blind Veterans Association Scholarship Program

This veterans group offers scholarships for blind veterans and their offspring. (See also *Blind Veterans Association*, page 303 and *Veterans Administration*, page 311.)

Website: https://bva.org/programs/scholarships

Phone: 1-800-669-7079

Christian Record Services

The Christian Record Services offers scholarships in all areas of study to undergraduate students who are legally blind.

Website: www.washington.edu/doit/christian-record -services-scholarship

Phone: 1-402-488-0981

Federal Student Aid

U.S. Department of Education's Federal Student Aid (FSA) office has a variety of information and resources available for blind and visually impaired students enrolled in education beyond high school.

Website: www.studentaid.gov

Phone: 1-800-433-3243

Fordham University Law School

Fordham University Law School offers the Amy Reiss Endowed Scholarship to students who are physically disabled and are interested in obtaining a law degree from Fordham Law School.

Website: www.fordham.edu/info/20645/financial_aid

Phone: 1-212-636-6815

Lavelle Fund for the Blind, Inc.

The scholarship is designed to help make quality undergraduate and graduate education affordable for U.S. residents who are legally blind, financially needy, and attending any of eleven selected private colleges and universities in New York State and Northeastern New Jersey.

Website: https://lavellefund.org/scholarship_program

Phone: 1-212-668-9801

Lighthouse Guild

The Lighthouse Guild offers up to twenty scholarships to college-bound high school seniors and at least one qualifying graduate student who are legally blind.

Website: https://lighthouseguild.org/support-services/academic-and-career-services/scholarships

Phone: 1-212-769-7801

National Federation of the Blind Scholarships

Each year, this organization supports scholarships for visually impaired students through each state's organization. It is the largest program of its kind offering some $250,000 each year for scholarships and awards to students in every state, including the District of Columbia and Puerto Rico. For more information about these awards and your state's organization, visit their website. (See also *National Federation of the Blind*, page 308.)

Website: https://nfb.org/programs-services/scholarships-and-awards/scholarship-program

Phone: 1-410-659-9314 x2415

Western Michigan University

Under the WMU Department of Blindness and Low Vision, a limited number of grants for financial support and scholarships are given out to graduate students. These students are then required to become employed after graduation in vision rehabilitation for two years for every year that financial support is provided.

Website: www.wmich.edu/visionstudies/scholarships

Phone: 1-616-387-3455

EDUCATION FOR VOCATIONS & INDEPENDENT LIVING

There are also national programs that are funded by donations from citizens and non-governmental programs. They offer opportunities for socializing, learning, and mentoring. Many of the large non-profit organizations listed in *Resources* under GENERAL, FINANCIAL & SOCIAL SERVICES on page 300 can provide the names of programs designed to help those with low vision and blindness to live more independent lives.

In addition, there are many schools for the blind and visually impaired located throughout the U.S. and Canada. The names and contact information for these schools can be found at the following website: www.teachingvisuallyimpaired.com/schools-for-the-blind.html

Clovernook Center for the Blind and Visually Impaired

Located in Cincinnati, Ohio, the Clovernook Center is designed to enable those who are blind and visually impaired to lead active, productive, and independent lives by providing employment, enrichment and recreation programs, and support services. (See also *Braille Printing House*, page 328.)

Website: https://clovernook.org

Phone: 1-513-522-3860

Hadley School for the Blind

The Hadley School is the world's largest educator for the blind and vision-impaired. It is conducted online, serving some 10,000 students. This online school offers courses on various topics such as technology, independent living, business, and leisure. Students can learn at their own pace and receive feedback from instructors.

Website: https://hadleyhelps.org

Phone: 1-800-323-4238

Helen Keller Services for the Blind

This organization supports early intervention for visually and hearing-challenged children, vocation training, and programs for senior citizens using cutting-edge technology and hands-on learning. This group operates schools largely located in New York City.

Website: https://www.helenkeller.org

Phone: 1-516-465-1234

Perkins School for the Blind

Perkins School for the Blind is the oldest school of its kind in the U.S. It services students who are blind, visually impaired, and deaf-blind from ages 3 to 22. It prepares children and young adults with the education and skills they will need to realize their full potential. Their teachers help them access core academics and address the social and independent living skills they will need. Perkins also offers a host of other services including diagnostic evaluations, transition programs, and Perkins' e-learning program for teachers of students with visual impairments.

Website: https://www.perkins.org

Phone: 1-617-924-3434

GUIDE DOG PROVIDERS

Guide Dogs for the Blind (GDB)

Located in San Rachael, California, this guide dog school prepares guide dogs to help empower individuals who are blind or visually impaired. GDB receives no government funding and there are no costs for individuals who receive a guide dog. Donors contribute through general contributions, bequests, grants, memorial and honor donations, charitable remainder trusts, and other planned giving options.

Website: https://www.guidedogs.com

Phone: 1-800-295-4050

Guiding Eyes for the Blind

Located in the New York townships of Yorktown Heights Patterson, and White Plains, this non-profit organization raises, trains, and socializes guide dogs to become guide dogs for the blind. There are no costs for individuals who receive a guide dog. They are 100% philanthropically funded by individual donors, general contributions, bequests, and grants.

Website: www.guidingeyes.org
Phone: 1-800-942-0149

Leader Dogs for the Blind in Michigan

Located in Rochester Hills, Michigan, this organization believes that everyone deserves a life of independence and mobility. All of their services are provided free of charge to their clients, including travel in the U.S. and Canada, room and board, equipment, and training. This means that no one is excluded from living their most fulfilling life due to lack of funds.

They are 100% philanthropically funded by individual donors, Lions Clubs, corporate partners, and foundations.

Website: www.leaderdog.org
Phone: 1-248-651-9011

Pilot Dogs

Located in Columbus, Ohio, Pilot Dogs was established to provide expertly-trained guide dogs, orientation and mobility training, and other valuable services free of charge to those who are visually impaired or blind allowing them to live with greater independence, safety, and mobility.

Website: www.pilotdogs.org
Phone: 1-614-221-6367

The Seeing Eye

The Seeing Eye is a philanthropic organization located in Morristown, New Jersey. Its mission is to enhance the independence, dignity, and self-confidence of blind people through the use of Seeing Eye dogs. In pursuit of this mission, The Seeing Eye:

- Breeds and raises puppies to become Seeing Eye dogs;
- Trains Seeing Eye dogs to guide blind people;
- Instructs blind people in the proper use, handling, and care of the dogs; and
- Conducts and supports research on canine health and development.

Website: www.seeingeye.org

Phone: 1-973-539-4425

FINANCIAL AID FOR ASSISTIVE PRODUCTS

Several national organizations listed under GENERAL, FINANCIAL & SOCIAL SERVICES beginning on page 300 also offer financial aid for assistive technology aids to those who are vision-impaired or blind.

Free White Cane Program

One of the National Federation of the Blind's purposes is to distribute free white canes for the blind. In fact, since 2008 they have given 100,000 free white canes to blind persons. To sign up for a free white cane, go online to the Free White Cane Program and complete the application, or call the NFB.

Website: https://freecane.nfb.org

Phone: 1-410-659-9314 and then press 7

I Can Connect

The *I Can Connect* program, which is also called National Deaf-Blind Equipment Distribution Program, is a federal and state program that provides free equipment and training for those with both significant hearing and vision loss who meet federal income guidelines. The program provides a variety of tech devices such as smartphones, tablets, computers, braille devices, and more. It is administered by your state where you reside. You can visit their website to find your state contact to apply.

Website: www.icanconnect.org

Phone: 1-800-825-4595

National Deaf-Blind Equipment Distribution Program

The National Deaf-Blind Equipment Distribution Program, which is also called *I Can Connect* program, is a federal and state program that provides free equipment and training for those with both significant hearing and vision loss who meet federal income guidelines. (See *I Can Connect* listing above.)

National Library Service for the Blind and Physically Handicapped (NLS)

This free service sponsored by the Library of Congress provides books and magazines in audio and braille formats, as well as a free player to listen to them. You can access the materials by mail or by downloading to your device. (See also *BARD*, page 302 and *National Library Service for the Blind and Print Disabled*, page 308.)

Website: www.loc.gov/nls

Phone: 1-888-657-7323

MANUFACTURERS OF ASSISTIVE TECHNOLOGY & ADAPTIVE SOFTWARE

The manufacturers below are listed under their specialties. This should provide a good starting place when looking to purchase any of these assistive products, however, you can also find additional products listed within the *Catalogs of Low-Vision Products* list found on page 335.

Additionally, many of these companies may have a dealer located near you, so that you may be able to see their products in person before deciding to purchase. Some of their products may also be available in the offices of low-vision optometrists, state rehabilitation centers, and/or VA Blind Centers. To learn more about any product, simply go to the manufacturer's website or contact the company directly for more information.

ASSISTIVE PRODUCTS FOR THE HOME

ADT Medical (On-Person Alarms)

The company's products detect falls. It can be worn as a pendant around the neck or on the wrist. It can work in the home and outside. The user can speak directly through the alarm

Phone: 1-855-499-0280

Website: www.adt.com/cf/bps/health

Bay Alarm Medical (On-Person Alarms)

The company's products detect falls. It can be worn as a pendant around the neck or on the wrist or as a smart watch. It can work in the home and outside. The user can speak directly through the alarm

Phone: 1-877-522-9633

Website: www.bayalarmmedical.com

Bureau of Engraving & Printing (BEP) (Money Reader)

This U.S. Bureau, under its U.S. Currency Reader Program, provides free money readers. To be eligible, you must show that you are legally blind and/or visually impaired, and that you are a U.S. citizen or national resident. Applications can be found on the website below.

Phone: 1-844-815-9388

Website: www.bep.gov/services/currency-accessibility/us-currency-reader-program

Cirbic.com (Watches, Clocks, and Scales)

Produces a wide range of products designed for those visually impaired. These include watches, clocks, and scales.

Website: www.cirbic.com

CVI Medical Equipment (Hospital Beds)

CVI produces a hospital bed that is voice-activated. Through voice commands it can allow you to raise and lower the head, foot, and overall height of the bed. Models are available for one person or for two.

Website: https://cvimedical.com

Phone: 1-214-363-2289

ECOVACS DEEBOT (Vacuums)

ECOVACS produces the DEEBOT vacuum cleaner. This vacuum cleaner can be programmed to operate on its own,at certain times, be voice-activated, and repower itself. It can also be hooked up to work with Amazon Alexa, Google Assistant, or Apple HomeKit.

Website: www.ecovacs.com/us/deebot-robotic-vacuum-cleaner

Phone: 1-844-326-8227

Flexabed (Hospital Beds)

Flexabed produces hospital-like beds for home healthcare that are voice-activated. Through voice commands it can allow you to raise and lower the head, foot, and overall height of the bed. Models are available for one person or for two.

Website: https://flexabed.com

Phone: 1-877-993-3710

GE Appliances (Air Conditioners, Espresso Machine, Dishwashers, Laundry Appliances, Mixers, Ovens, Ranges, Refrigerators, Ventilation, Water Heaters)

This company manufactures products that allow users to control their GE smart appliances from their phone or other smart devices. GE has a wide range of smart products. Their controls are integrated to work with Google Assistant and Amazon Alexa.

Website: www.geappliances.com/ge/connected-appliances

Phone: 1-800-626-2005

Govee (Lighting)

This company produces a wide range of smart lighting devices for the home including indoor and outdoor lighting, light strips, lamps, and smart bulbs.

Website: https://us.govee.com

Phone: 1-855-925-3570

iRobot (Vacuums)

iRobot produces the Roomba vacuum cleaner. This vacuum cleaner can be programmed to operate on its own, at certain times, be voice-activated, and repower itself. It can also be hooked up to work with Amazon Alexa or Google Assistant.

Website: www.irobot.com/en_us/roomba.html

Phone: 1-866-747-6268

KOHLER (Touchless Faucets)

KOHLER produces a line of smart touchless faucets that can be turned on and off by motion movement, along with its speed of flow and temperature. Not only does this provide a hands-free process, it is also hygienic.

Website: www.kohler.com/en/products/kitchen-faucets/shop-touchless-kitchen-faucets

Phone: 1-800-456-4537

LG ThinQ (Dishwashers, Laundry Appliances, Ovens, Ranges, Refrigerators, TVs, and Vacuums)

This company manufactures products that allow users to control their LG smart appliances from their phone or other smart devices. Their line of products include refrigerators, ranges, ovens, dishwashers, laundry appliances, vacuums, and TVs. Their controls are integrated to work with Google Assistant and Amazon Alexa.

Website: www.lg.com/us/lg-thinq

Phone: 1-800-243-0000

MEDICAL GUARDIAN (On-Person Alarms)

The company's products detect falls. It can be worn as a pendant around the neck or on the wrist. It can work in the home and outside. The user can speak directly through the alarm.

Phone: 1-800-910-5056

Website: www.medicalguardian.com

Oratell (Hospital Beds)

Oratell produces hospital beds that are Alexa voice-controlled. Through voice commands it can allow you to raise and lower the head, foot, and overall height of the bed.

Website: www.oratell.com/product-category/alexa-bed

Phone: 1-801-615-2322

SwitchBot (Curtain Controls, Door Locks, Lighting Controls, Vacuums, and Window Blinds)

This company produces a wide variety of smart devices including curtain controls, door locks, lighting controls, vacuums, and window blinds.

Phone: 1-855-696-0888

Website: https://us.switch-bot.com

tado (Heating and Cooling Products)

This company produces smart heating and cooling management products for the home. The tado app allows users to adjust temperatures in their home. Their products can also work with Google Assistant, Amazon Alexa, and Apple HomeKit.

Phone: 1-415-301-3525

Website: www.tado.com/all-en

Verilux (Lighting)

Verilux lamps and bulbs provide users with a full spectrum of light inside their homes. The lights in their lamps can be dimmed or brightened, which can reduce eyestrain. Their products have been designed to promote feelings of well-being and enhance focus.

Phone: 1-800-786-6950

Website: https://verilux.com

BRAILLE PRODUCTS

HIMS Lifestyle Innovation

This company specializes in highly rated portable braille products. All products carry a factory warranty, a 30-day money back guarantee, and tech support.

Website: https://hims-inc.com

Phone: 1-888-520-4467

Braille Printing House

Located in Cincinnati, Ohio, the Clovernook Center's Braille Printing House produces braille reading material for individuals, libraries, and global consumers. They produce textbook materials, tactile graphics, periodicals, calendars, menus, business cards, instruction manuals, medical documents, and more. (See also *Clovernook Center for the Blind & Visually Impaired*, page 319.)

Website: https://clovernook.org/braille-printing-house

Phone: 1-513-522-3860

HumanWare

This company has many products for totally blind consumers including braille embossers (braille printer), portable braille display tablets, braille displays for computers, handheld audio book players, and a portable text-to-speech reader (OCR). They also have a full line of desktop low-vision machines and portable magnifiers. All products carry a factory warranty, a 30-day money back guarantee, and tech support.

Website: www.humanware.com/en-usa/home

Phone: 1-800-722-3393

MAGNIFICATION/READING PRODUCTS

Dolphin Computer Access

Dolphin produces adaptive software such as SuperNova, Easy-Reader App, and ScreenReader. They have strong technical support and offer training on their products through video tutorials and user manuals.

Phone: 1-866-797-5921

Website: www.yourdolphin.com

Enhanced Vision

Enhanced Vision is a leading developer of low-vision devices for the visually impaired including macular degeneration, glaucoma, cataracts, retinitis pigmentosa, and diabetic retinopathy. Low-vision assistive technology enables people to read, write, and fully participate in life. Enhanced Vision has brought many of the industry's most innovative assistive technologies to the market.

Website: www.enhancedvision.com

Phone: 1-800-811-3161

Freedom Scientific

Freedom Scientific designs and manufactures devices that are intended to promote independence, allowing blind and low-vision individuals the same access to information as their sighted peers. This includes software products such as ZoomText, JAWS, Fusion, and OpenBook. Freedom also offers desktop and portable video magnifiers, such as the Topaz OCR desktop as well as refreshable braille displays that connect to computers.

Website: www.freedomscientific.com

Phone: 1-800-444-4443

HumanWare

(See *HumanWare* for more information regarding their desktop low-vision machines and portable magnifiers, page 329.)

Low Vision International (LVI)

LVI sells video magnifiers, reading machines, and magnifying lamps. They also offer complementary items, such as software and tools, to make the workplace more ergonomic. All products carry a factory warranty, a 30-day money back guarantee, and tech support.

Website: www.lviamerica.com

Phone: 1-888-781-7811

NonVisual Desktop Access (NVDA)

NVDA is a screen reader software product that enables blind or visually impaired people to access information on a computer. NVDA is bundled with eSpeak, a free-speech synthesizer.

Website: www.meinnvda.de

Phone: 1-408-418-5610

Ocutech

Ocutech produces bioptic telescopic glasses for those with visual impairments. It combines a telescopic device with conventional glasses to help people see things that are at a distance more clearly. They are essentially small binoculars worn on or above regular eyeglasses.

Phone: 1-800-326-6460

Website: www.ocutech.com/resources/about-bioptics

Optelec

Optelec's goal is to help those in need who are coping with vision loss. Their products include daily living aids, PowerMag handheld magnifiers, electronic video magnification, and audio solutions. They are designed and built to help people lead independent and full lives.

Website: www.optelec.com

Phone: 1-800-444-4443

Vispero

The Vispero family of companies include Optelec, Freedom Scientific, and Enhanced Vision. Vispero is an American company that provides a full range of low-vision hardware such as the Topaz CCTV, Ruby portable electronic magnifiers, ClearView CCTV, Merlin CCTV, ONYX CCTV, and many more low-vision options.

Freedom Scientific provides industry leading JAWS (Jobs Access With Speech) screen-reading software, ZoomText magnification software, and Fusion software that combines both products into one software package. Warranties and tech support are included in their price. Local dealers provide local assistance including demonstrations, sales, and support as needed.

Website: https://vispero.com

Phone: 1-800-444-4443

Zoomax

Zoomax specializes in portable electronic magnifiers and desktop video magnifiers. They also offer low-vision e-glasses. All products carry a factory warranty; a 30-day money back guarantee; and tech support.

Website: www.zoomax.com

Phone: 1-866-887-6565

MEDICAL AIDS

MedReady, Inc.

MedReady provides medication dispensers. They have enlarged trays to hold more medications. They have made their tray removable, and added a rechargeable battery pack to safeguard against power outages. This also means MedReady can be used on short trips, eliminating the confusion of a suitcase filled with different pill containers.

Phone: 1-310-328-7557

Website: www.medreadyinc.net

Omnis Health

Omnis Health provides high-quality diabetes testing supplies, including the Embrace family of blood glucose monitoring products. Produces Embrace Talking Blood Glucose Monitoring System.

Website: www.omnishealth.com

Phone: 1-877-979-5454

Prodigy

Prodigy produces affordable, high-quality, easy-to-use products with a focus on the low-vision and blind diabetic patient. This includes the Prodigy Autocode Talking Blood Glucose Monitoring Kit.

Website: www.prodigymeter.com

Phone: 1-800-366-5901

SECURITY DEVICES

Arenti

Arenti produces smart indoor and outdoor cameras, pet cameras, and baby monitors.

Website: https://arenti.com

Phone: 1-866-999-7866

Eufy

Eufy produces smart devices for home protection. This includes door locks, security cameras, and alarm security sensors.

Website: https://www.eufy.com

Phone: 1-800-988-7973

Lockly Vision

By combining a smart lock with HD video doorbell, users can Verify visitor identities, have conversations, and even remotely unlock the door through the live stream on the Lockly App, no matter where you are.

Website: https://lockly.com/products

Phone: 1-669-500-8835

SwitchBot

This company produces a wide variety of smart devices including door locks, curtain controls, vacuums, window blinds, and lighting controls.

Website: https://us.switch-bot.com
Phone: 1-855-696-0888

Vivint

Vivint produces smart devices for home security including doorbell cameras, outdoor cameras, door locks, and car and garage alarms.

Website: www.vivint.com
Phone: 1-855-592-1297

THERMOSTATS

Ecobee Smart Thermostat Premium

This thermostat comes with a large LCD display. It has an internal sensor that balances temps in your home, and it has a built-in smart speaker for use with Alexa or Siri systems. Temperature displays can be set in Fahrenheit or Celsius readings.

Website: www.ecobee.com/en-us/smart-thermostats
Phone: 1-877-932-6233

Electeck Digital Thermostat

These room and/or house thermostats come with a large easy-to-read backlit LCD display; however, it is not voice-activated. Models are available in programmable and non-programmable units, and they can work on electric or gas systems. Temperature displays can be set in Fahrenheit or Celsius readings.

Website: https://electeck.store/products

Emerson Sensi Smart Thermostat

This thermostat comes with a large LCD display. It works with many home automation and voice-control platforms, including Amazon Alexa, Google Assistant, Apple HomeKit, and Samsung SmartThings. Temperature displays can be set in Fahrenheit or Celsius readings. Settings can be changed by using its free app.

Website: https://sensi.copeland.com/en-us/products/wifi-thermostat

CATALOGS OF LOW-VISION PRODUCTS

American Printing House for the Blind (APH)

The American Printing House for the Blind sells low-vision materials, educational material to assist with early childhood development, and products associated with core curriculum through high school. APH offers catalogs for products, parts, and press books on demand.

Website: www.aph.org
Phone: 1-800-223-1839

HearMore, Inc.

HearMore offers products for those with hearing impairments and low vision.

Website: www.hearmore.com
Phone: 1-800-881-4327

Independent Living Aids

Independent Living Aids sells products related to low vision and blindness, healthcare, daily living aids, mobility, durable medical equipment, assistive technology, and hearing.

Website: www.independentliving.com
Phone: 1-800-537-2118

LS&S: Learning, Sight & Sound Made Easier

This catalog has many aids for education, lighting, and living aids for low-vision customers. These include items for entertainment and electronics, magnification products, lighting and lamps, basic living, and so on. You can go to their website and view their catalog.
Phone: 1-800-468-4789

MaxiAids: Products for Independent Living

The MaxiAid catalog has a large selection of helpful products for the blind and visually impaired, including braille items, canes, calendars, talking watches, computer products, magnifiers, music players/recorders, specialty sunglasses, and much more. If you call, you can request a free catalog be sent to your home. Or you can go to their website and view their catalog.
Website: www.maxiaids.com
Phone: 1-800-522-6294

About the Authors

Laura J. Stevens, MSci, received her master's degree in nutrition science from the Department of Nutrition Science at Purdue University in West Lafayette, Indiana. Since graduation, she had worked at Purdue as a researcher who investigated the relationship between diet and health disorders. As an author of nine successful books on diet, behavior, and allergies, Laura now deals with low vision herself. She lives with her amazing cats, Bentley and Seis, in Lafayette, Indiana.

Thomas Blackman, MHA, received a master's degree in Blind Rehabilitation from Western Michigan University. Thomas provided Orientation & Mobility instruction at Bosma Enterprises in Indianapolis for several years. He then served as Founder and Director of the Assistive Technology program at Easter Seals Crossroads beginning in 1988. In 1998, he formed EYE Can See, Inc. in Indianapolis, which continues to provide adaptive hardware and software products for blind and low-vision customers in Indiana and Kentucky. Thomas currently resides in Westfield, Indiana.

Index

OTHER SQUARE ONE TITLES OF INTEREST

$16.95 • 192 pages • 6 x 9-inch paperback
ISBN 978-0-7570-0501-5

YOUR GUIDE TO UNDERSTANDING, IDENTIFYING, & OVERCOMING THE PROBLEMS CAUSED BY INCORRECT GLASSES, POOR LIGHTING, NIGHTTIME GLARE, COMPUTER SCREENS, AND SO MUCH MORE

WHAT YOU MUST KNOW ABOUT EYESTRAIN

JEFFREY ANSHEL, OD
BESTSELLING AUTHOR OF SMART MEDICINE FOR YOUR EYES

$16.95 • 144 pages • 6 x 9-inch paperback
ISBN 978-0-7570-0479-7

CHOOSING A SAFE COURSE OF ACTION THAT WORKS FOR YOU

WHAT YOU MUST KNOW ABOUT DRY EYE

HOW TO PREVENT, STOP, OR REVERSE DRY EYE DISEASE

JEFFREY ANSHEL, OD
BEST-SELLING AUTHOR OF SMART MEDICINE FOR YOUR EYES

$17.95 • 288 pages • 6 x 9-inch paperback
ISBN 978-0-7570-0449-0

CHOOSING A SAFE COURSE OF ACTION THAT WORKS FOR YOU

WHAT YOU MUST KNOW ABOUT

AGE-RELATED MACULAR DEGENERATION

HOW YOU CAN PREVENT, STOP, OR REVERSE AMD

JEFFREY ANSHEL, OD
LAURA STEVENS, M.Sci

$16.95 • 176 pages • 6 x 9-inch paperback
ISBN 978-0-7570-0410-0

A PRACTICAL GUIDE TO SUPPLEMENTS, DIET, AND LIFESTYLE FOR PEAK OCULAR HEALTH

WHAT YOU MUST KNOW ABOUT

FOOD AND SUPPLEMENTS FOR OPTIMAL VISION CARE

OCULAR NUTRITION HANDBOOK

JEFFREY ANSHEL, OD
Best-selling Author of Smart Medicine For Your Eyes

For more information about our books, visit our website at www.squareonepublishers.com